FATIGUE FREE
Made Crystal Clear!

My Sounds Increase Your Life-Force Energy

DAWN CRYSTAL

outskirts press

DEDICATION

This is for all those who suffer from excessive fatigue, and who know the answer is not drugs. There are alternative drug-free methods to relieve fatigue that are safe, effective, and rapid. It takes some guidance and an open mind to obtain the possibilities of these non-traditional methods, including mine. Let's enhance your energy reserves!

Table of Contents

FOREWORD

Dawn is a pioneer of voice-sound-energy relief of pain, anxiety, fatigue. She makes life-enhancing sounds with her voice, a gift she discovered as an adult. She has done this for over 20 years, with individuals or groups.

She has been rich and has been homeless, energetic and fatigued, and she discovered she had a gift in using her voice to relieve herself and others of troubling conditions, like pain, fear, and fatigue

She now has a sophisticated web site, DawnCrystalHealing.com. Dawn feels a Higher Power has guided her to go Internet, go global. She started from nothing, "heart-guided."

Who does she think should seek help? Anybody. Everybody. People who have tried everything else: holistic, natural, traditional. She's had success with a wide variety of problems: fear, pain, and fatigue. She has helped herself and others to find happiness.

The multitude of testimonials to the effectiveness of her technique demonstrate something beneficial is happening. We know that mind and body are interconnected. Hypnosis and auto-suggestion can produce dramatic changes, including pain and fear relief. Many medical successes are attributed to the "placebo effect," where belief in the likely efficacy of a cure helps produce a cure. Voodoo curses can cause the believers great harm. Human attraction, "animal magnetism," can make us feel better when we are ill or hurting. Faith healers have some surprising results, too. However it does so, Dawn's gift works, and there are those who are witnesses to its effectiveness.

Discussing her techniques with Dawn, I found that her description of moving energy throughout the body and overcoming blockages resembled the techniques I learned years ago of auto-suggestion, self-hypnosis, in which progressive relaxation is produced by visualizing a warm, relaxing wave traveling through various parts of your body, starting with your feet. I have first-hand knowledge that such techniques worked for me, including relieving occasional tension headaches and facilitating falling asleep.

Those who would like to hear Dawn talk about herself and her techniques are invited to listen to this 25-minute interview done in August 2018, https://www.talkshoe.com/conf/summary/4977560.

I have been pleased to help get Dawn's story into print as her writing coach and editor. Another kind of personal change occurred: her energy and optimism have been infectious!

Douglas Winslow Cooper, Ph.D.

douglas@tingandi.com

WriteYourBookWithMe.com

Walden, NY

Fall 2019

ACKNOWLEDGMENTS

First, and once again, I thank my coach and editor, Douglas Winslow Cooper, Ph.D., without whom this book would never have been written.

My editor and I thank Cheryl C. Cohen, Director of Membership at Greater Monroe Chamber of Commerce, for her skilled editorial assistance.

My dog, Hoku (Hawaiian for "star"), brings me daily joy and peace and deserves my gratitude. I can't imagine my life without him.

Disclaimer

The information in this book is not intended to be a replacement or substitute for medical advice. It does not diagnose, treat, or cure medical conditions. Please see a medical professional if you need help with such problems.

PREFACE

I wrote this book because I wanted everyone to know that there is hope for becoming free of excessive fatigue, naturally, fast, easy, and effectively.

You should read this book if you are suffering from continuing fatigue or you know someone who is, and you or they have tried many different techniques without success to get relief.

I am known by many for my healing vocals. I offer my sound healing sessions with a loving heart by phone and in person.

Especially relevant to overcoming fatigue is my Unlimited Energy Series:

https://dawncrystalmaui.clickfunnels.com/package-a22871798

Don't miss it!

Dawn Crystal

DawnCrystalHealing@gmail.com

Maui, Hawaii

Fall 2019

Prologue: Overcoming Fatigue

"Fatigue makes cowards of us all." – Vince Lombardi

"The first virtue in a soldier is endurance of fatigue;
courage is only the second virtue." – Napoleon Bonaparte
[funny-quotes-life.com]

"Fatigue makes fools of us all. It robs us of our skills, our judgment,
and blinds us to creative solutions." – Harvey Mackay
[azquotes.com]

If we are to live successful, courageous, happy lives, we must learn to overcome fatigue. Part of defeating fatigue is recognizing and avoiding its causes.

I'll start by excerpting / quoting some material from an excellent article in WebMD.com [https://www.webmd.com/balance/how-tired-is-too-tired#1] that helps us identify when our fatigue is out of the ordinary:

How Tired Is Too Tired?

Do you feel like you're always tired? …when you suffer from a constant lack of energy and ongoing fatigue, it may be time to check with your doctor.

What Is Fatigue?

…lingering tiredness that is constant and limiting…. You may be too exhausted even to manage your daily affairs.

Allergies, Hay Fever, and Fatigue

Symptoms: Fatigue, headache, itchiness, nasal congestion, and drainage

…. One way to reduce symptoms of allergic rhinitis -- including fatigue -- is to take steps to avoid the offending allergen.

Anemia and Fatigue

Symptoms: Fatigue, dizziness, feeling cold, irritability

[Anemia] affects more than 3 million Americans. For women in their childbearing years, anemia is a common cause of fatigue.

To confirm a diagnosis of anemia, your doctor will give you a blood test.

Depression, Anxiety, and Fatigue

Symptoms: Sadness, feeling hopeless, worthless, and helpless, fatigue

.... you might be in a depressed mood most of the day. You may have little interest in normal activities. Along with feelings of fatigue, you may eat too much or too little, over- or under-sleep, feel hopeless and worthless, and have other serious symptoms.

Although the specific causes of depression and/or anxiety are unclear, these are highly treatable medical problems. Medication, psychotherapy or a combination of the two can help relieve symptoms.

FIBROMYALGIA AND FATIGUE

Symptoms: Chronic fatigue, deep muscle pain, painful tender points, sleep problems, anxiety, depression

....one of the more common causes of chronic fatigue and musculo-skeletal pain, especially in women. Fibromyalgia and chronic fatigue syndrome are considered separate but related disorders. They share a common symptom -- severe fatigue that greatly interferes with people's lives.

FOOD ALLERGIES, FOOD INTOLERANCE, AND FATIGUE

Symptoms: Fatigue, sleepy, continually exhausted

Although food is supposed to give you energy, new medical research suggests that hidden food intolerances -- or allergies -- can do the opposite.

HEART DISEASE AND FATIGUE

Symptoms: Fatigue with an activity that should be easy

If you find yourself becoming exhausted after an activity that used to be easy -- for example, walking up the steps -- it may be time to talk to your doctor about the possibility of heart disease, the leading cause of death in women.... medication or treatment procedures can usually help correct the problem, reduce the fatigue, and restore your energy.

RHEUMATOID ARTHRITIS AND FATIGUE

Symptoms: Fatigue, morning stiffness, joint pain, inflamed joints

[Rheumatoid arthritis] is another cause of excessive fatigue...early and aggressive treatment is the best approach....

SLEEP APNEA AND FATIGUE

Symptoms: Chronic fatigue, feeling exhausted upon awakening, snoring.

According to the National Sleep Foundation, more than one-third of adults in the U.S. snore at least a few nights a week. If snoring is associated with periods when breathing stops, a condition called "sleep apnea," a person may have daytime sleepiness and excessive fatigue.

If left untreated, sleep apnea can increase your risk of stroke or heart attack.

TYPE 2 DIABETES AND FATIGUE

Symptoms: Extreme fatigue, increased thirst and hunger, increased urination, unusual weight loss.

.... lifestyle measures are important in staying well with type 2 diabetes. They include smoking cessation and blood pressure control, and reduction in cholesterol.

Underactive Thyroid (Hypothyroidism) and Fatigue

Symptoms: Extreme fatigue, sluggishness, feeling run-down, depression, cold intolerance, weight gain.

The problem may be a slow or underactive thyroid.

According to the American Thyroid Foundation, approximately 17% of all women will have a thyroid disorder by age 60.

Blood tests known as T3 and T4 will detect thyroid hormones. If these hormones are low, synthetic hormones (medication) can bring you up to speed and you should begin to feel better fairly rapidly.

If you have one of these medical conditions, then you need to confer with a medical professional.

On the other hand, many people have non-medical causes of excessive fatigue, and these people are candidates for the kind of sound-energetics work that I do. My techniques can also support medical therapies, if used.

Editor Marcia Angell commented on the people who are seeking help from alternative therapies:

"You see that the people who are drawn to alternative medicine are often fairly healthy and they go to alternative medicine for what I call the 'symptoms of life.' Fatigue, joint pains, inability to concentrate, perhaps, the kinds of things that anyone over twenty-five gets at some point." [https://www.brainyquote.com/quotes/marcia_angell_526879]

Chapter 1

CAUSES: ENERGY DRAINS

"A significant part of personal energy management
involves protecting ourselves against anything (or anyone) that can drain our vital energy force, commonly
referred to as 'energy drainers."
– Seline Shenoy, author and coach.

AUTHOR AND COACH Seline Shenoy listed six major "energy drainers"
for us to avoid:

1. Toxic People: *A person is considered toxic if they perpetually disre-*
spect, abuse, belittle or criticize you....

2. Unhealthy thought patterns: *Every single thought and belief car-*
ries a specific energy pattern. When we succumb to negative self-talk

and other unhealthy thought patterns subject ourselves to undue anxiety, worry and stress....

3. Neglecting your body's needs: When we neglect to meet our bodies' basic needs such as good nutrition, regular physical activity and getting sufficient sleep, we could potentially face serious health consequences....

4. Living an inauthentic life: When we live our life as sell-out — that is, we live a life that isn't in alignment with our authentic self and the values that we cherish — we can feel extremely fragile on the inside....

5. Living in a stressful environment: You may not realize it but your environment has a significant impact on your comfort levels. A noisy, messy or stressful setting can totally sap your energy....

6. Unexpressed emotions: A significant energy drainer is unexpressed emotions that we have repressed over prolonged periods of time. When we allow unpleasant feelings like guilt, shame, anger and resentment to fester within us, it can eat away at our spirit and deplete our sense of inner peace....

[http://thedreamcatch.com/energy-drainers-that-are-slowing-you-down/]

With regard to the company we keep, Meiyoko Taylor wrote [in everydaypowerblog.com] that we must avoid three types of **energy-draining people**:

1. **"Drainers** are constantly buried in chaos and drama, then they come to you to feed off your positivity. They are physical, emotional, and mental vampires."

2. **"Complainers** are toxic people who never take responsibility

     FATIGUE FREE MADE CRYSTAL CLEAR!

for their actions. They just drain energy from those around them."

3. **Shamers:** "Out of all three toxic people, this type is the most harmful to your personal and professional growth. A shamer is always trying to look down on everything you do, think, or say. No matter what accomplishment you achieve, they try to mock you and make you feel inadequate."

Chapter 2

WORK

Look at a day when you are supremely satisfied at the
end. It's not a day when you lounge around doing
nothing; it's when you've had everything to do, and
you've done it.
- Margaret Thatcher, former British Prime Minister

WORK CAN BE tiring, but the achievement it produces can re-energize us! It has been said, "work is love made visible." It is love made real.

"Our fatigue is often not caused by work, but by worry, frustration, and resentment." – Dale Carnegie

"Happiness does not come from doing easy work but from the afterglow of satisfaction that comes after the achievement of a difficult task that demanded our best." – Theodore Isaac Rubin

[brainyquote.com]

At home and sometimes in the workplace, **work is love made real**. We work to support ourselves and others and we offer goods and services that this work produces. We want to do this effectively and efficiently, without letting fatigue keep us from our goals. As Dale Carnegie noted, fatigue may not come from our efforts but from the attitudes we bring to the job.

As psychologist Rubin notes, successful completion of something hard brings an afterglow, like winning at a game.

But the **work must have a purpose.** French poet/philosopher Albert Camus wrote about the punishment that the ancient gods gave to Sisyphus: *The gods had condemned Sisyphus to ceaselessly rolling a rock to the top of a mountain, whence the stone would fall back of its own weight. They had thought with some reason that **there is no more dreadful punishment than futile and hopeless labor.*** Without a purpose, work leads to the resentment that Carnegie identified.

As I grew up in my poor family, a welfare family, I knew from an early age that I'd have to work. My first job was as a nine-year-old with my own newspaper route. It was survival! I feared that if I did not work, I'd be poor for the rest of my life.

From teenage years on, I always worked. I missed being a kid, really. As I grew up, my jobs got better, from waitress to marketer and then law enforcement, followed by having two beauty businesses. I always worked hard, often volunteering for overtime.

But this made me tired. Drained. Sick some of the time, too much of it, really. My immune system was not getting enough sleep.

Now I know that I have to listen to my body, paying attention to fatigue. Sometimes I turn down opportunities to make more money. I no longer work myself to the bone. I manage my energy to avoid crashes. No longer a workaholic, I am taking care of my body, my brain, my energy.

Recently, I worked with "Joe," a big-time East Coast lawyer who got my Unlimited Energy Program from a telesummit. We had a 30-minute session.

"What shall we work on, Joe?"

"I almost never listen to these telesummits, but I'm glad I did. I am in my mid-50s, pretty well-known. I'm busy. Lots of clients. Beautiful wife. Lovely home. Great kids. However, my wife is a high-maintenance woman, which means I've got to continue to find the Next Big Case. I cannot afford to slack off."

"I understand."

"Yes, I am doing what I was born to do, but these long trials really tire me out, and I have to keep myself going with caffeine, grabbing quick lunches, eating on the go. It's a daily drain from 7 a.m. to 9 p.m. or so, and then I have to work on the week-ends. My wife and I are addicted to this income, which means I must keep running."

I could feel the strain he is under. "Take three deep breaths, Joe."

He hardly knew how to do that.

I started making appropriate sounds for a couple of minutes. "Joe, how so you feel now?"

"A bit more relaxed."

I made more sounds. "Imagine a Divine Light above your head. Move your disturbing energy to this region. You must move the energy from other people out of you, so you are feeling your true self."

More sounds. "How about now?"

"I feel unusually peaceful."

"Keep clearing the energy from other people. Have you always had to work, work, work, work?"

"Yes, and my dad was this way, too."

"Your body needs a break. I will help you work in a more steady, grounded way. Can you clear this belief system you got from your father and replace with a belief that you can be effective in a steady way, not so stressful?"

"I can try that."

His father's influence was great, but as a child Joe missed his father's support.

More sounds from me helped him clear this belief system. "Your dad was too caught up in his own run-run-run belief system."

I had Joe continue deep breathing, as I made more clearing sounds.

"How do you feel now?"

"Oh, my God, I feel like a new person. I've never felt this way before! I can see the world around me clearer. I've never even been able to take a deep breath before."

"I will restore your own life-force energy."

"I don't understand, but I trust you."

I grounded him and his life-force energy for a couple of minutes.

"Now, Joe, breathe deeply again."

"I never felt this way, with much less weight. I even feel I can see more clearly. I don't need my contacts! I am amazed at what you have done in 30 minutes."

Before we parted, I advised him to place boundaries around himself to protect from the energy of others in the courtrooms.

He thanked me profusely, "I feel like a new person!"

We are lucky to have work we like, but it is easy to over-do it, too. Maintaining a balance between your career work and your personal life is essential to happiness and to keep from burning out due to fatigue.

Chapter 3

Running a Business

Running your own business does not mean that you have lesser things to do or a shorter to-do list than you had when you were employed. When you think about it, entrepreneurs get stressed out from the moment they start planning the business until the time that they are exiting it."

Here are four approaches, quoted from this article, for combating boss-fatigue. [http://www.smbceo.com/2011/05/17/entrepreneurial-fatigue/]

1. Hire an assistant.

2. Look to your friends and family for support.

3. Join local communities of like-minded individuals so you could share experiences, ask questions, and get advice

4. Find your own happy place.

Each of these will take some effort, investment likely to pay off. One reader of the article, David Cameron, added, "Excellent advice, from my experience as well. Working solo definitely has its ups and downs and I have sought to balance my life by doing other things like singing and golf. I return refreshed and ready for the next challenge."

Using my voice-sound technique, I have helped numerous business executives overcome fatigue and become more energetic.

Before I write about someone else, let me tell you more about myself. For years, in my second marriage, I owned two beauty businesses, which I started from the ground up, without prior experience.

I owned a tanning salon, which we had in an historical building, which we remodeled. I got little help from my drunk of a second husband. I really needed a second employee. In the first year, the tanning salon, I had one employee and did all the paperwork, barely paying myself anything.

Opened a second salon, 50 miles from my house, a big mistake. I hired some employees, people I did not know well, and my living situation was dicey, too. I became overworked. Even so, the salon succeeded for a while, without a manager other than myself. Money seemed to leak out. The second marriage was in crisis, pulling my attention from my businesses. I was spread too thin, and the business failed.

The marriage failed, too.

I closed both businesses, but in retrospect, I think the first one could have survived, if I had not opened a second one too soon. I should have kept my ego under control and not started a second shop too soon.

Sometimes, you get tempted to over-do it, and I over-did it, but I learned from it.

    FATIGUE FREE MADE CRYSTAL CLEAR!

Here is an example of my work with one of my clients.

"Jasmine" had been married to a wealthy man. That marriage failed. A second marriage failed as well. She tended to be pushy. Being a beautiful, exotic woman, she used that.

She ran two businesses and was a mother to three kids. Her two ex-spouses were not supporting the lifestyle she sought. Added to that, she often exercised strenuously to keep up her good looks.

She asked me to help her have more balance in her life.

"You are kind of taking on the weight of the world," I commented, noting that her shoulders and neck were stiff. "You've got two businesses, three kids, no nanny, and the ex-spouses are not helping enough."

"I'm forced into this. I need the money, but I don't know how to change this situation."

"Your higher self tells you to get more help…get a nanny, get the exes to pay more or help more. This problem is coming from your ego, thinking you can do it all. You have a lingering cold, and you need to give yourself some TLC, some Tender Loving Care. Why not rent out some of your living space? You'd ease your income problem. You are not using the whole house."

"Yes. I'm going to do both, rent out a room, and hire a nanny."

She had a breakthrough, in coming to trust having someone help care for her kids. Her distrust had come from her childhood experiences.

I made my sounds. "Push this old energy, these old beliefs, to a light over your head, and release them. Now, ground your life-source energy through your feet."

I asked her permission to end with a heart-opening activation, to help her trust more, and be open to abundance.

"Yes, please do that heart-activation."

When I finished, I asked her how she felt.

"Thank you, Dawn, I feel so much better, like a million bucks! I am going to make some changes, especially finding a nanny I can trust."

She left, obviously happier and more peaceful.

I understood Jasmine's difficulties. Like Jasmine, I had a life period during which I had to handle everything without help. I ran myself ragged.

Being a middle child, just as I had been, Jasmine had gotten less attention from her parents, and, just as I had, she also had an emphasis on trying hard to look good. She was trying to do too much on her own.

Based on our session, Jasmine planned to increase her income by renting out part of the large house she owned, and she decided to get some help with the children.

Both moves required trusting others. The rule is to trust but verify, make sure those you rely on are worthy of that trust. If the people are trustworthy, these changes will relieve much of the fatigue caused by trying to do too much by oneself.

Chapter 4

Spouses

Confession of a Relationship Counselor (Celeste)
[http://www.marriagelaboratory.com/blog/
fatigue-the-common-enemy-of-a-happy-marriage/]:

"Because I like you, I'll let you in on a little secret . . . sometimes Rich and I fight.... These fights range in subject matter from very serious issues like finances and parenting techniques to sometimes even more serious issues like what's the most effective way to keep our kitchen sponges from stinking? .... I've noticed one common theme throughout almost all of them – fatigue. **Fatigue!** The Common Enemy of Marriage. It is out to get yours like a monster in the night."

She cites several studies that conclude that sleep deprivation is a major cause of such fatigue, and she offers some practical suggestions, which we quote:

1. *Go to bed earlier.*

2. *Frequently acknowledge the real source of your emotions to yourself and your spouse.*

3. *Don't keep sleep score. [One is deservedly more tired than the other....]*

4. *Fake it till you make it. [Do your best without excuse.]*

5. *Do not make tired a way of life.*

6. *Prioritize – put the best things first.*

For many years, I drained my life energy. It had happened when I dated. It happened in my marriages. I was too needy, not having been loved as a child, and I kept looking for a father-figure. Even others who saw my strengths tended to drain me. The energy they saw eventually became my healer energy. My second marriage was especially a big drain, as living with an alcoholic for years exhausted me. Finally getting away energized me. I learned from this we have to be willing to sever some connections. Once I did that, I found my own power. I found a gift that allows me now to help others break free, too.

Despite following sound advice, some spouses are still going to find themselves overly fatigued. Using my voice-sound technique, I have helped them re-energize. Here's an example.

"Mertha" just met with me over Skype. She's living in the UK, in an island offshore. Despite this scenic location, she feels stuck, finds she cannot move forward. Why? Her husband of many years has just gotten out of alcoholic rehab. He used to be successful, but no longer is.

   FATIGUE FREE MADE CRYSTAL CLEAR!

Mertha started right in, "I feel I'm stuck on this island. I no longer love him. He's kind of controlling. I feel drained."

"For how long has this gone on?" I asked.

"As long as I've known him."

"Do you want to know why?"

"Sure."

"Your husband is riding on your coattails, dragging along behind you, using your energy, taking it from you. He's been doing this for many years."

"Well, I'm sick of it. I often have to leave the house. I feel trapped. Even though he is working on planning a new business, I think we've stagnated. I need for us to improve our finances. I like my job, but it is not enough for me to live on my own."

I shared my own experience from living on this beautiful Hawaiian island, "You have a higher cost of living being on an island. You may need to move and to downsize. You will need to find your kind of work elsewhere."

"I cannot wait for his venture to pay off. Frankly, I fear he may go back to drinking."

"I'm going to make my clearing sounds, to cut the energy cords binding you to needy people." I made my voice-sounds and had her take a few deep breaths. "How do you feel now?"

"A lot better, freer."

I made some sounds to relieve her of the fear she could not make it on her own. I encouraged her to be self-sufficient.

"Mertha, how do you feel now?"

"Expanded in my heart. I can take on the world. My chattering mind is quiet."

I made more voice-sounds and encouraged her to continue to seek another place to live and work.

"That's what I need to do. Wow! That's a big shift in my life with just a thirty-minute session. I feel we have made a breakthrough, and I can take my first steps in a new direction."

Clearly, she has a substantial distance to travel, but she is off to a good start.

You have to see the truth about your life. When much younger, I too lived in a fog, so I understood how Mertha was not seeing her true abilities, not realizing she could flourish on her own. Part of what I do with people is to show them the truth, help them find their gifts and their happiness and use my voice to free their blocked energy and overcome fatigue.

Chapter 5

PARENTING

PARENTING COUNSELOR ERIN Schlicher wrote, "The fatigue that can come with motherhood or fatherhood (whoever is doing the primary amount of parenting) is certainly not glamorous or boast-worthy, but it is a legitimate daily struggle for many of us. It should be said that there is a range of different types of exhaustion. The spectrum includes—but is not limited to—physical exhaustion, feeling burnt out, bored, frustrated, and a feeling of being defeated or fed-up."

[https://www.empoweringparents.com/article/
im-so-exhausted-4-tips-to-combat-parental-burnout/]

She offered the following practical tips:

1. Be a **"good enough"** parent.

2. Find **support**.

3. Expand your **toolbox.**

4. Recognize and **focus on the positive**.

Schlicher quoted **Mother Teresa**: "Do not think that love, in order to be genuine, has to be extraordinary. What we need is to love without getting tired."

I never have been blessed with children of my own, even though I thought in my first marriage that I would have children. My husband's becoming blind put an end to that. The second marriage, the "rebound" one to the drunk, was clearly not a good place into which to bring a child, and fortunately we did not.

I have expressed my maternal side with my pets, my "fur babies," dogs and cats. I love them deeply and treat them very well. When we can, my Hoku and I go for long, relaxing Maui walks. So, I have some sense of what being a parent is like.

I talk to my dog, and I swear he smiles at me sometimes when I do. I have cared for many homeless cats. I have my car partly filled with food for them, share it as I walk, and they greet me. Some other people now seem to be following my example where I live.

I have worked with many parents who found their energies seriously depleted in dealing with the tasks associated with parenting.

I worked with a lady, "Emily," who bought our Unlimited Energy program from a telesummit. She, too, lived on Maui, as I do now. She later moved to California. Her thirty-minute session focused on her five children.

A very attractive woman, Emily easily married wealthy men, and these

                    FATIGUE FREE MADE CRYSTAL CLEAR!

five children were from five different men. They were sort of a cash crop.

"These relationships never worked out. I had thought these men would contribute more to the raising of the children. I ended up working hard cleaning houses to supplement the child support, and not all five men have come through with what they owe."

The children ranged from four years old to twelve. She would have someone watch the kids while she exercised to work on her looks and her figure.

"I love my children, but raising them alone is a real chore."

I had met her in person. "I see you've had some cosmetic surgery, and you are busy with your cleaning service, and I get the sense that you are afraid that others will cheat you, especially your husbands."

"Yes, I saw cheating as a child. I was the fifth of six kids, hoping to get attention from a dad who was an alcoholic, whom I often had to try to get to come home from the bar. I decided I would have to manage my own life all on my own.

"You came to believe you were not going to get support, and now you would like help, help you had not looked for before."

"Right."

I made my sounds and redirected her life force energy.

"How are you feeling?"

"Calmer. My mind has stopped racing, I have not known before how to quiet it."

"You feel you have the weight of the world on your shoulders, with no one you can trust. I myself had much the same experience. Do you feel you have a Creator you can ask for help? If you do not pray, can you meditate a few minutes a day?"

"Yes, I could do that."

I worked more on her lack of trust and her need for support. "Do you have digestive issues? Constipation?"

"Definitely."

"After our session, you will find you have relief from these problems." I did another ten minutes of sound therapy. "How do you feel now?"

"I feel more optimistic. I can see 'outside the box' I have put myself in."

I encouraged her to work on herself daily, to make time for herself, and do some meditating. She agreed to do this.

Interestingly, I could see her face was so much more relaxed right after the session…and this made her even prettier.

She thanked me warmly for our session.

I find that my parent-clients are often stressed out by raising their kids. They get relief from our sessions. They need to step back sometimes from being parents and focus on their own needs, using daily ten-minute meditations and some regular exercise. I encourage them to calm their racing minds and tune into their heartbeats and their breathing.

　　　　　　　　FATIGUE FREE MADE CRYSTAL CLEAR!

Chapter 6

SLEEPLESSNESS

"As a **survivor** of Post-Traumatic Stress Disorder (PTSD), I understand overwhelming stress and the **anxiety and sleeplessness** that result from living with it. I understand that **stress is an elusive and ever-changing opponent.**

"That's why it's important to have **multiple things to try** until you find the right solution for you at the right time. Knowing that there are practical stress hacks in this book that you can turn to means you'll have a **closet full of tips** at your disposal." – Michelle Whitney, author of *Stress Hacks: 166 Tips and Tricks to Free Yourself from Stress and Sleeplessness and Reclaim a Relaxed Life.*

An older book that offers sleep-time help is by Barbara L. Heller, M.S.W., *How to Sleep Soundly Tonight: 250 Simple and Natural Ways to Prevent Sleeplessness.*

Depending on whether there are some techniques mentioned in both books, you have in them some 250 to 416 ways suggested for dealing with sleeplessness. My voice-sound technique provides yet another approach, one which some have found quite effective.

I went for several years with severe stress from my first husband's blinding eye injuries and having to live with his mother. I hardly slept, it seems. We had moved to the U.S. East Coast, just getting by on his disability payments, awaiting the results from a medical malpractice suit. His life had been destroyed by his blindness. I was a nervous wreck, taking care of him and trying to pay the rent. We were battling with lawyers, tearing our marriage apart. Love had gone down the drain. At one point, I went for a month without sleeping. I knew this was dangerous.

No conventional sleep aids helped me. However, the crises led to a small spiritual awakening. I went to some spiritual retreats. They did help. I learned from my teachers, gained spiritual insight, which much later became my voice gift.

We fought for my husband's rights, and we won. Eventually, I aligned with my soul, and my ability to sleep returned. I made a successful body-mind-spirit connection, grounding my energy, gaining balance, stability and peacefulness. This experience has helped me to help others around the world.

Today, I had three different clients, and each had some sleep disorder. I'll describe one of them.

    FATIGUE FREE MADE CRYSTAL CLEAR!

I worked with Arati, who had bought a new program of mine, Healthy Joints, that includes a session with me. We got on the phone, together:

"Hi, Dawn. Actually, I bought your Healthy Joints program, but I have another issue I thought you could help me with. I am 80 years old, and I've had difficulty sleeping all my life."

"That can be very disturbing. Are there any traumas you can identify from your earlier years?"

"Ten years ago, my son was on drugs, rampaging through our house. That was difficult to deal with. Many years before that, my parents had been in Germany and they were supporters of the Hitler regime, the Nazis."

"Wow! How did they treat you?"

"They were rally rather distant, distracted by their Nazi activities. The energy throughout Germany at that time was disturbing. My childhood was quite upset. We were on a war footing. I did try to guard myself. Most of the people I encountered had poor relationships with me."

"You picked up on the violent energy of Germany at that time, and it has been carried along within you all these decades. You heard about some terrible things, even as a child, whether you remember them or not."

I made my sounds and they started to move the blocked energy that was keeping her from trusting others. Her neck and shoulders showed extreme tautness, tension, that slowly lessened. I understood why my Healthy Joints program appealed to her.

"Ever since I was a child, I heard nighttime sounds that made me afraid…not so long ago, I was hearing my son disrupt our home in the night…. I thought you could help me."

"You need to stop blaming yourself. Your son is responsible for his drug problem. Your husband was not much help in bringing him up. Fortunately, your son seems to have been turned around recently."

"Yes, he has outgrown his rebelliousness."

We worked to clear the blocked energy from her body. She was tense, wound up, on edge. As I vocalized, I could see she was changing.

"How are you feeling now?"

"Better, I am even starting to yawn."

I took that as a good sign. "Is that unusual?"

"I never yawn."

As I made more of my special sounds, I could see her relaxing further.

After more sound-grounding her to the Earth, I asked, "How are you feeling now? We worked on many issues."

"Well, I am yawning now. A good sign. I haven't yawned in years. I had gotten your Joint Health session, and I am finding myself changed."

After our session was over, I told her, "Arati, let me know how you make out. Send me an email." I'm looking forward to hearing from her.

Many people are disconnected within their body-mind-spirit. Their Higher Self, their Soul, needs to be freed from the unconscious belief systems that they picked up from their early environments. We work

    FATIGUE FREE MADE CRYSTAL CLEAR!

to clear these harmful patterns. These thoughts can run through their minds like a computer do-loop, repeating over and over. Clearing these thoughts produces relaxation and freedom from the chattering mind. This can make a huge shift even in these short, 25-30-minute sessions, which is surprising and rewarding, with results that are long-term, lasting, cumulative.

Chapter 7

OBSESSIONS

FEW MENTAL STATES are as tiring, as fatiguing, as Obsessive-Compulsive Disorder, OCD. The patient repeats the same actions over and over again.

A fine self-help book on OCD has been written by Edna B. Foa and Reid Wilson, *Stop Obsessing! How to Overcome Your Obsessions and Compulsions.* The book is described as follows, "Once considered almost untreatable, OCD is now known to be a highly treatable disorder using behavior therapy. In this newly revised edition of *Stop Obsessing!* Drs. Foa and Wilson, internationally renowned authorities on the treatment of anxiety disorders, share their scientifically based and clinically proven self-help program that has already allowed thousands of men and women with OCD to enjoy a life free from excessive worries and rituals."

Alternatively, one suffering from OCD might find it more effective, and less unpleasant, to work on this problem with me, using my voice-sound-therapy techniques.

I was one of these OCD people early in my life. As a poor teenager, I worked several jobs to get money. I needed to be in control. Money was an obsession. I took on more work than I could handle, despite being pretty much the caretaker in our family, giving help and advice to all. That seemed to be "my job," to be a surrogate mother, even to people older than I. I extended myself way outside my comfort zone.

In school, I had learning difficulties, partly due to exhaustion because I took on so many responsibilities. I had a form of OCD. I am happy not to be plagued by OCD now, and I do enjoy helping people who come to me now for our sessions. I guess I always will be this way.

Working on myself now, I find I can manage my time better, filter out what is not important, and handle my life more efficiently. I make my free time "sacred time." I relax to restore a balance in my life. I like helping others to reach this pleasurable state.

As you might expect, OCD individuals often need more than one session to overcome their compulsions. One client, call her "Meghan," I've worked with over a decade. She's younger than most of my clients, now in her thirties. She's a wise "old soul" in a pretty, young body. She reminds me of how I was. We both grew up amid the chaos of a dysfunctional family, including having a brother with a mental disorder.

She's not really heavy, but she has been obsessed with her weight. We worked on it for a while, helping to get her over bulimia, her eating and then throwing up. We resolved her anorexia, perhaps caused by having been sexually abused by a babysitter in her youth.

A yoga teacher, Meghan is very health conscious, quite alert to maintaining proper exercise and diet. If anything, you might think she is too thin. (I know the saying that a woman cannot be too rich or to thin, but I don't agree.) She is lovely, but does not believe it. Why?

Perhaps because her father left her mother (and thus Meghan, too) for a younger woman. Both mother and Meghan wanted her father's affection, without getting it.

Her mother eventually remarried. Meghan's step-father was a political activist, in his case, a compulsion of sorts, as well. This only confounded her upset. Her boyfriends tended to be users/losers, because she felt unworthy of a better partner and did not require respect from the ones she got.

Meghan and I worked on these issues for years. I would clear her during our sessions, with lots of emotion, but the problems recurred, requiring many sessions. We unpeel her OCD onion of layers of obsessions and problems, primarily over weight and over money. She has overcome bulimia and she has gained a distance from her conflicts with her step-father.

Her OCD symptoms have included working obsessively, some of which was strictly psychological, some of which she had to do financially. By helping her overcome her childhood trauma, we found for her a better work-life balance and even discovered some activities that would bring her more income for less time invested.

Some clients require multiple sessions, as some problems are very deep-seated. Some clients bring memories of past lives, and we deal with genetic and historical inheritances. I am familiar with the need to handle one layer at a time, as I had to do with myself.

Meghan is an example of a woman who had many experiences in this life, and perhaps in a past life, experiences that have shaped the person she is today. She has learned to cope with these experiences in a way that allows her to live in the present more fully and less compulsively.

Part of my work with certain clients is to bring them up to the present, so that they are more aware of the here and now.

Chapter 8

NEWS AND POLITICS

"**Politics Fatigue Syndrome** — it strikes many people in many ways. Swelling anger. Watery expectations. Sniffling insecurity. That nagging sense of hopelessness when it comes to the efficacy of political action.

"Historically, one of the salient symptoms is extreme lethargy. A while back, a reporter from the *Atlanta Constitution* noted that there was not much interest in the congressional elections in New Hampshire: 'The people are utterly tired of politics.' The year was 1877." Linton Weeks, *The Protojournalist*, NPR July 25, 2014.

[https://www.npr.org/sections/theprotojournalist/2014/07/25/334101621/the-diagnosis-politics-fatigue-syndrome]

LINTON WEEKS CITES some statistics to show that political fatigue is not new, though the 2016 presidential election seems to have increased it. Diana L. Banister, a political strategist, is quoted as finding four causes:

1. Widespread malaise.

2. Misguided media.

3. Disgust with the process.

4. Disillusionment with politicians.

None of these is likely to change soon, so if you are suffering from political fatigue, you may find a session of voice-sound therapy just what you need.

> "If you feel like there is too much news and you can't keep up, you are not alone. A sizable portion of Americans are feeling overwhelmed by the amount of news there is, though the sentiment is more common on the right side of the political spectrum, according to a Pew Research Center survey conducted from Feb. 22 to March 4, 2018." [https://www.pewresearch.org/fact-tank/2018/06/05/almost-seven-in-ten-americans-have-news-fatigue-more-among-republicans/ft_18-05-17_newsfatigue_7-in-10_exhausted/

A majority of those polled by Pew regarding the 2016 presidential election felt themselves victims of "information overload."

Concerning political news, 77% of Republican-leaning people found themselves "worn out" versus 61% of those who leaned toward the Democrats. Some of the difference might be due to the generally more negative coverage of President Trump than of his Democrat critics. Of the respondents 71% of the women reported themselves "worn out" by the news, and 64% of the men held that view.

Two centuries ago, American Poet William Wordsworth (1770-1850) wrote, "The world is too much with us;" he needed a break!

Sometimes we have to turn off the television, silence the radio, ignore the banner headlines on newspapers and magazines, and recover from information overload, news fatigue. I myself don't spend much time with such concerns, such drama. When I have a client with this problem, I find my sounds help clear the mental clutter and promote a calm, more rested condition.

A client, we'll call her "Holly," I have worked with for several times a year for several years. She grew up in a politically active U.S. East Coast family. Especially her father expressed strong views often. She was exposed to them from childhood. She moved to Hawaii a few years ago. This area is beautiful and more peaceful, but she is very interested in environmental issues, about which she is easily stressed.

Her new home community is definitely upscale, with beautiful vistas, and the people are quite sensitive to environmental issues, being very rich and wanting to live in the nicest surroundings. Unfortunately, such issues come into play almost every November, at election time. I could see this in a pattern as to when she needed my help.

Her beliefs about being very connected with the Earth made her very vulnerable to any proposed environmental changes at election time. If her candidate lost, she really needed help to calm her chattering mind

   FATIGUE FREE MADE CRYSTAL CLEAR!

To calm her, I would talk with her, and then I would give her a session with my reassuring sounds. Fortunately, she is very responsive, becoming less upset. I think she needed to overcome a habit that started with her father's strong opinions being often expressed during her childhood.

Working with her has helped. She is doing better at election times, without being as upset. She says she sees a Divine Power in action, and she is more willing to accept what comes.

A lot of people at election times get "nerved up," picking up the energy that comes through the media and "mass consciousness." They would do better to expose themselves to less media, and they can keep up by reading only a modest amount of news and commentary.

Chapter 9

FRIENDS

TO HAVE A friend requires being a friend, and often that means stepping up and giving compassion to one you care about. In return, however, you may find this draining, rather than energizing. There has been much written about "compassion fatigue." A recent article by Jennifer Koza listed five major ways in which you can become aware your caring has become wearing:

1. APATHY: YOU LITERALLY CAN'T ANYMORE

"If you find yourself feeling apathetic toward a person you know is in an unhealthy relationship, then this may be the first sign of fatigue. Stepping away from the situation (at least for a little) and asking for help from a trusted friend or counselor may be the best thing for you at this time."

2. ANGER: You're Angry at the Person Experiencing Abuse

"Sometimes, it's easier to get angry at your friend instead of the root of the problem: their partner who is doing unhealthy or abusive things to them. Just keep in mind that they are going through a lot with the relationship."

3. ISOLATION: You're Avoiding People

"If you find that you are not just avoiding the person in an unhealthy relationship, but also everyone in your life, then you may be experiencing compassion fatigue."

4. NEGATIVITY: You've Become a Pessimist

"A significant negative change in your normal behavior can be a sign of compassion fatigue."

5. FATIGUE: You're Tired All. The. Time.

"… when you're experiencing compassion fatigue, the exhaustion is overwhelming."

What does she suggest you do about this?

Be Honest with Yourself and Others

"Often compassion fatigue is a result of either forgetting to check-in with yourself or knowing how you're feeling, but not being open or honest about it. Sometimes it just feels easier to put other people's needs before your own. However, **we can't actually be there for others if we aren't there for ourselves first."**

[https://www.joinonelove.org/learn/5-signs-youre-experiencing-compassion-fatigue/

Those employed in the various helping professions are particularly susceptible to compassion fatigue. A new book by two such clinicians offers help: "Those in the helping professions are constantly at risk of compassion fatigue, yet many have little guidance on how to deal with it effectively. A fresh workbook approach for compassion fatigue, burnout and stress, providing all the tools you need to leave work at work - and let it go." The book is *Overcoming Compassion Fatigue: A Practical Resilience Workbook, Kindle Edition,* by Martha Teater and John Ludgate.

Sometimes, unconventional approaches, such as mine, can prove helpful in overcoming the tiredness, the fatigue, one experiences when trying to aid one's friends and family.

I wish I had a story about friends in my life, but as a child I was so different and surrounded by such a dysfunctional family that I had no friends in my childhood. It was sad, but it made me stronger. Even now, I have only a few friends, but those I have I cherish. One of them is quite furry, a handsome dog, and I have a lot of good times with him. I do know that some people are energized by their friendships but others find these relationships quite draining.

Today I had a client, "Cathy."

She had bought my anti-aging package, but I asked her what she really wanted to work on. Sometimes, clients have a more pressing need.

"I see age spots developing, and I look like my mom. I am tired."

I asked, "What would you most like to discuss? Let it be of your own free will."

She indicated that being tired was the big issue.

"How long has your energy been drained?"

"For a while."

"Are you married?"

"Yes."

"How is your marriage?"

"Fine."

"What can you tell me about your childhood?"

"It was not too good, as I did not have a loving dad. He was an absent alcoholic. Mom was more of a girlfriend than a mother."

"Are you an over-achiever?" I was picking this up from her energy. "Do you go above and beyond?"

"Yes. That could be a problem."

"Without having had a caring father around, you could have been feeling the need to try hard to gain your father's love."

"Yes. I over-achieve. I have lots of friends, but I have these high expectations on myself, and some of them I actually have achieved. My friends expect much help from me. I give advice and I help to the point of forgetting about my own well-being. I have a friend whose house I am checking on daily and caring for her cats…it's a twenty-mile round-trip. For another friend, I drive forty miles round-trip several days a week to check up on the landscaper. I used to like writing and some other activities, but I am so busy helping my friends, I am exhausted, driving all over the place. I have committed to do too much for these pals of mine!"

"We have to erase the belief that you have to please other people, as you hoped to please your father. You are knocking yourself out with these activities in addition to your career. You have to overcome this impulse."

"You have hit it right on the head. I feel responsible."

"All the heavy weight of the world on your shoulders is going to be taken away." I made some sounds. "Breathe deeply. How are you feeling now?"

"Better. I must have been breathing very shallowly, because this deep breathing is making me feel different."

I continued sound-therapy. "Are you ready to release this feeling of widespread responsibility?"

"Yes, I am ready."

I made some more sounds. She started to cry in relief, not a sad cry, but a happy one. She was breaking up her cemented belief system.

"How do you feel now?"

　　　　FATIGUE FREE MADE CRYSTAL CLEAR!

"My head is clear, and my mind is no longer going in 100 directions."

"Yes, we are clearing these old belief systems, having these disturbing energies flow from you to your feet and into the ground."

Thirty minutes had gone by quickly. I wanted to give her guidance for the future. "Think about what has brought you joy in the past, and do more of that. Perhaps write down more of your poetry or even write a book."

"Thank you! I feel like a million bucks. I have never felt this calm in my life."

Cathy's story is a common one. Many of my clients try too hard to please people, because they, as children, did not get the attention and love they sought. Our inner child needs to have such beliefs purged.

I have found that a simple thirty-minute session, because I can pinpoint these false beliefs easily, clears these harmful energies and allows my clients to make new and better choices for themselves to change their futures dramatically. These old compulsions are removed, cleared, and the client is freed from them.

Chapter 10

———⚬———

HEALTH

A RECENT ARTICLE by Amanda Gardner, "9 Health Conditions that Could be Making You Tired" [https://www.health.com/anemia/fatigue-causes] offers details on the following disorders that are not simply the result of burning the candle at both ends:

1. ANEMIA

"Anemia means you don't have enough red blood cells to take oxygen to all the distant outposts of the body. Less oxygen means lower energy and more fatigue."

"The most common form of <u>anemia</u> occurs when you're low in iron, which, in turn, could be the result of gastric bypass surgery, heavy periods, chronic diseases, or vitamin deficiencies."

To treat this successfully, you need the proper diagnosis from a medical professional.

2. **CELIAC DISEASE**

"Celiac is an autoimmune disease that causes the immune system to attack the small intestine when a person eats gluten, a protein found in wheat, rye, and barley."

"The only treatment is avoiding foods that contain gluten."

3. **SLEEP APNEA**

"It's when your airways close and you actually stop breathing repeatedly during the night, which, needless to say, wakes you up pretty quickly. Because of those frequent disruptions, people with sleep apnea walk around exhausted."

"The go-to treatment … is a continuous positive airway pressure (CPAP) device, which keeps the airways open while you sleep. CPAP machines work, but many people don't like wearing them…. The only actual cure for sleep apnea is losing weight or surgery to remove tissue from your throat."

4. **CHRONIC FATIGUE SYNDROME**

"It's fatigue that lasts for at least six months, that gets worse with mental or physical exertion, and that doesn't get better no matter how much you rest. It's more common in women in their 40s and 50s."

"There's no cure for the condition or even a specific treatment. Instead, lifestyle measures like pacing yourself can give you more energy. Some people benefit from medication or cognitive therapy."

5. FIBROMYALGIA

"Fatigue isn't the most pronounced symptom … but it's a big one, along with poor-quality sleep and memory and mood problems."

"While there's no cure, a variety of medications can help control <u>fibromyalgia symptoms</u>. Exercise, relaxation, and stress-reduction measures also may help."

The most pronounced symptom is pain, and some pain-killers and anti-depressants are helpful.

6. CHRONIC PAIN

"Being in constant pain–for any reason–will tire you out."

"Contact your doctor to see if there's a way to treat the underlying condition causing the pain while also addressing that tired feeling."

7. THYROID PROBLEMS

"Both an underactive and an overactive <u>thyroid</u> can cause fatigue. The more common culprit though is an underactive gland…."

An underactive thyroid gland produces "hypothyroidism."

"Hypothyroidism is treated with replacement thyroid hormone."

8. DEPRESSION

"Fatigue due to <u>depression</u> is more than just a lack of energy going about your day; it's also apathy, problems focusing and remembering, and feeling overwhelmed and unmotivated."

"And some antidepressants may make it worse…. explore non-drug treatments like cognitive behavioral therapy."

9. Multiple sclerosis

"The fatigue of multiple sclerosis, a chronic disease that damages the nerves, can have several different causes, some of which would exhaust anybody."

"Then there's lassitude, a type of fatigue that only people with MS get. This so-called 'MS fatigue' is more severe, usually happens every day, gets worse with heat and humidity, and can come out of seemingly nowhere."

"Talk to your doctor about treatments for MS and treatment for specific symptoms including fatigue."

Some of these conditions are not likely to be relieved by my techniques: anemia, celiac disease, sleep apnea, fibromyalgia, thyroid disorder, and multiple sclerosis need other treatments. How about chronic fatigue, chronic pain, and depression? These conditions would seem possible to improve by my voice-sound techniques. When I work with a client, I don't start with a diagnosis, I just do what I can do, and we see whether we get improvement. Usually, we do.

Here's an example. I worked with woman with chronic fatigue. Anna, living in Italy; she found me because of her fatigue, a very common complaint of my clients.

I had not worked with her before, but she had followed me on telesummits, having heard me on live calls on that show. She decided to take the plunge and buy a package.

Anna runs a business, has been married 13 years, following an earlier divorce. The second marriage has gotten a bit stale, and their financial problems play a role, keeping her from visiting her aging parents, whom she'd like to see and help more.

She has three teenagers from the first husband, who had turned out to be very different from what she had expected. They grew apart. Even though divorce is rarer in Italy, she knew she wanted to be happier and she could be.

"I love him dearly, more than he loves me. He's goal-oriented and not that good at managing money. I feel we are falling behind. It's not quite an equal partnership, and I am tired. Fatigue is affecting me thoroughly. Doctors have not been able to find the cause. It's a mystery. I have lots of good ideas, but I lack the energy to follow through. Do you see something?"

"It looks like you came from a big family. True?"

"Yes, I have eight brothers and sisters, most in Italy. We don't see each other as often as I'd like, partly because we are hustling in businesses. I want to work on this."

I noticed she was a bit high-strung, nervous, talking even faster than I was! "Let's find out why you are so wound up. How was your childhood?"

"Mom raised nine kids and did well by most of us, even the middle children like myself. I had a normal childhood, with a distracted but loving Dad. Good provider, and I knew I was loved"

"Your energy patterns show you have several friends. You like to help people, give them advice, give them a hand. You step up to the plate."

    FATIGUE FREE MADE CRYSTAL CLEAR!

"I do a bit too much of that, wearing myself out, rather than getting my stuff done. I am angry with myself for not setting and keeping boundaries."

"Your soul is telling you to change that, as you come into a new phase of your life in 2019, finding some new things to do, new directions, which may energize you." My sounds and sensing indicated she had many people connected with her, draining her energy. Sadly, her spouse was one of these major drains.

"I know people do drain me, but I don't know how to stop.""

"I'll show you. First, your health seems good, but keep in touch with your physicians. Breathe deeply, then exhale the non-productive elements into a white light above your head. Feeling lighter?"

"Yes."

"Anna, I see your energy being drained by people connected to your energy ports. Shall I disconnect them?"

"Yes."

I started disconnecting people from her energy ports. "Better now? With fewer disruptors?"

"I do feel lighter in my stomach. I have had digestion and constipation issues, as you guessed."

"You have these problems because of all these drains from your stomach area." I cleared more pathways along her meridians. I helped her body to retain beneficial energy. "How do you feel now?"

"I feel energized. I wasn't sure at the start that I could stay awake for my session. Now, I see a smile on my face in the mirror."

I gave her some suggestions about a morning routine to put a healthy boundary around her to protect her from potential draining by others.

"How are you doing?"

"Actually, I don't feel I have any remaining problems."

I grounded her life-force energy right to the ground.

She said she loved the session and would have another the next time she felt she needed it.

I do specialize in handling fatigue, a frequent complaint. Chronic fatigue has a variety of causes, not always done by others, but often so. The others are not trying to hurt us but they see our energy, are drawn to it, and then proceed to absorb and drain it from us. I am here to help people clear their traumas and keep them from losing energy and thus becoming fatigued. And we do it without chemicals! My clients learn how to do it for themselves by creating energy boundaries.

Chapter 11

DIETING

"Long-Term Dieting Can Cause Fatigue and
Tiredness

"Less food means less nutrient going into your body
and less energy availability.

"You're stuck between a rock and a hard place in a way
because you need to sacrifice calories in order to liber-
ate fatty acids from the fat cell. But the consequence is
that you might not have as much energy as you usually have.

"The result is that you can feel tired and lack that 'get
up and go' attitude you normally have."

[https://www.instantknockout.com/ik/
dieting-and-fatigue-the-relationship/

You can improve this somewhat by altering your food choices. Here are some foods that help restore your energy [https://www.healthline.com/health/food-nutrition/foods-that-beat-fatigue];

Unprocessed foods

Fresh, seasonal fruits and vegetables

Non-caffeinated beverages

Lean proteins

Whole grains and complex carbs

Nuts and seeds

Water

Vitamins and supplements

Bananas

Oats

Chia seeds

Furthermore, regular exercise will help build your endurance.

When I was a teenager, somewhat of an outcast, I deprived myself to try to maintain a very slender weight. I put my health at risk, trying to look good. From ages 14 to 18, I was pale, anemic, fatigued. My mother was too busy with her own issues. I was poorly supervised. A concerned neighbor, Pam, stepped in. She told me she knew our family was having difficulties, and she invited me to talk with her. Pam became almost a second mother to me during this time.

"You are too thin," Pam commented. She gave me food and advice on food, such as not to live only on raisins! I ate more wisely. My energy

                    FATIGUE FREE MADE CRYSTAL CLEAR!

increased. I became more comfortable with being a normal weight. Pam's kindness helped turn my life around. Perhaps that is one reason I am so eager to help others.

Some of my clients have come to me with fatigue problems that have responded well to my voice-sound treatment techniques. I also have a program on weight loss, Clear All Your Weight Issues Fast, with Sound Energy Clearance. Some of my phone sessions deal directly with such weight problems.

I worked with someone yesterday, a person who had bought one of my programs, and she brought up some issues not directly on the program topic. Penny is from the UK. She said she needed help with her joints.

"Hi, Penny. Thank you for buying my program. Thank you for trusting me to help. What do you want to work on?"

"I do have trouble with my joints. I'm in my 60s, and I have a lot of pain and fatigue. I have had a few accidents in my past. Now, I feel tired, off-balance."

"I understand. With your permission I'll scan your body. I can see the impact of having fallen off the horse. You worked for a while with a chiropractor. How do you feel?"

"Drained of energy. I'm always dieting, but I never lose weight. I keep hoping I will feel better. I need to do both: lose weight and gain energy."

"You are going in the right direction. At 62, you are showing some imbalance in your energy system. You are heavier than you want to be. You have people who are not respecting your boundaries, but are draining your energy. Do you often feel nervous? As though driving a car with one foot on the gas, one on the brake, and burning rubber."

"Yes, exactly. I'm stagnated."

"I expect that you are interested in moving to a new chapter of your life in retirement. What do you do for fun?"

"I hang out with my husband, who is not into the same things I am interested in. My family is not much interested either, so I have to hide my spiritual side. I want to become more outgoing and active."

"Penny, you're wise to be searching for good advice, but you have to take action on what you have already learned. You have to move on. Access your energy. Your metabolism has slowed, causing you to lose energy and adding weight. Your inner child tempts you to break your diet."

"Yes, I feel some days that I must have something more to eat, but I know I should not eat it."

I made some of my sounds and commented on her being "stuck," needing a new direction, perhaps a hobby. "Imagine a beautiful Divine Light and breathe into it."

Her energy was clearly stagnated. "Stay seated as I work to move your energy through the blocked regions in your joints and the rest of your energy system, while you breathe deeply…. How are you feeling?"

"Lighter, less drained."

"You have to be willing to reveal your true self to others, and you may find they love you." I made more of my sounds, then asked her to release the old thoughts, old beliefs. Ten minutes more of intense clearing were needed. She had systems I found to be unusually blocked.

"Oh, Dawn, your twenty-five-minute session has done more for me than any sessions I've had from others. I feel I have much more energy now to take action."

"Penny, thank you. You need to spend some more time daily listening to your own heart, to get beyond just listening to the mp3 recordings. If you do that, you will start to feel freer and you will gain added insight on what new direction you want to go."

"I will try, thank you for spending this special time with me. It seemed short, but may be life-changing."

Many of my clients have problems with lack of energy. They see me as a "mover and a shaker," getting them into motion. Penny needed clearing and encouragement to follow her true spirituality, even if others disagree.

These clients need to be able to "come out of the closet" and discuss their views with those close to them. Stagnation comes from fear, being unwilling to take the chances to be themselves. They have to have courage to change.

Like Penny, many clients have several issues they want addressed. In this case, weight, dieting, and fatigue all needed to be addressed for Penny to achieve a more active and fulfilling life.

Chapter 12

STRESS

OUR DAYS ARE filled with "stressors," events and situations which cause us to respond psychologically and physically. When they are scary, these can produce a "fight or flight" response, with our body preparing us to resist or to evade. As Rosie M. Spielman describes in her excellent text, *Psychology*, stress can be harmful or even beneficial when it impels us to do things which further our goals.

Negative stress occurs when we perceive a situation as harmful or potentially so. Positive stress occurs when we see an opportunity to achieve a goal.

For instance, an athlete improves performance under the stress of competition, at least up to a point, beyond which level of stress, performance actually deteriorates. Beyond the optimal level of stress, Spielman notes, people feel burned-out, "they are fatigued, exhausted, and their performance begins to decline. If the stress remains excessive, health may begin to erode as well."

One natural approach to reducing your stress hormone levels is to spend some time communing with nature: "Taking at least twenty minutes out of your day to stroll or sit in a place that makes you feel in contact with nature will significantly lower your stress hormone levels. That's the finding of a study that has established for the first time the most effective dose of an urban nature experience. Healthcare practitioners can use this discovery, published in *Frontiers in Psychology*, to prescribe 'nature-pills' in the knowledge that they have a real measurable effect." [https://www.sciencedaily.com/releases/2019/04/190404074915. htm?utm_source=dlvr.it&utm_medium=twitter]

Reducing your stress is not the only way to combat your fatigue, however. It won't surprise you to know that some of my clients come to me to have me use my voice-sound techniques to be re-energized, because they are suffering from fatigue.

I worked with a lady recently, Barbara, who had found me through a telesummit where she had bought several packages in the past. During the anti-aging program session with her, a woman in her 50s, it was clear she was coping with the results of three divorces and handling an important business.

"Hi, Barbara, its been about half a year since we worked on your pain. How are your hands and feet now?"

"They are doing better, but I have some other issues. My doctor is concerned that stress is harming my body, despite my working out a lot. I run a company and I try to reduce that stress with exercise."

"I'll look at your energy. Yes, you do have a stressful job. I'm picking up that you are working out too much, to the level that you are developing stress injuries from exercise."

"Yes, though they are improving, with your help. My doctor says my blood sugar and hydration are low."

"Let's dive right into it."

"I work out seven days a week."

"That may be excessive. I feel that you are over-doing it. You can choose to cut back or not. Your health issues are telling you something. You are overdoing it. You need to cut back on the running. Seven days a week and several times some days is too much."

"You can see that?"

"Yes, your inner child is asking you to take breaks, to relax to read a book. You are overdoing it."

"I want to look good. My failed marriages have made me feel unworthy."

"You are a powerful woman and have a right to have high expectations. But, again, you seem to be trying too hard, and you are not the twenty-year-old you once were."

"You nailed it. My father, as you guessed, was never around, leaving me feeling abandoned by him. My mom was a bore. My dad died in his forties, and I did not have his attention, even though I competed with my older sister to get it. You are right. I am really tired. You've spotted it. Do what you can to clear me of this compulsion."

"First, we have to replace this feeling of not being good enough. You must drop this, give your body time to recoup." I made my special sounds. "Relax your shoulders and back and legs, and let your energy

     FATIGUE FREE MADE CRYSTAL CLEAR!

flow to the ground, draining the stress that comes from your job and your expectations. Take deep breaths. Are you feeling better?"

"I'm starting to relax more, and starting to breathe more deeply than I usually do."

"You were not aware that you had a pattern of shallow breathing. Are you ready to drop this effort to please your father, who passed away years ago?"

She started to weep.

"What are you feeling?"

"I've been walking around with the load of not being loved. As a child I did not understand my dad was trying to provide for his family, and I mistook it as his not wanting to be with me."

I made some more sounds, and I could hear her crying.

"How are you feeling now?"

"Sadness and frustration are leaving me, and I am feeling a bit lighter. This session is deeper than ones I've had before,"

I kept working on Barbara's pain, including her feet and ankles…and her aching legs.

"Do you feel better?"

"Yes, I know I was ready for this session. You hit it on the head. It was not only my job, but my body, stressing me out."

"Cut back on your exercising. Do it three times a week to give your body time to recuperate. Reward yourself with treats when you have done a successful exercise session."

"Yes, I'll do that. I have been denying myself some chocolate doughnuts. You have told me something others did not recognize. I will cut back on the exercise and pick up a non-stressing hobby. I'll schedule another session in with the future."

This reminds me a lot of myself growing up. I was an over-achiever as a child, even at as young as age nine, competing for my dad's attention. I worried a lot about my looks and ran myself ragged to look good. My alcoholic dad did not give me attention; he did not know how to do better. I would sit with him at the bar to try to get him leave the bar… even when I was as young as nine. He would get more drunk, leaving me sad and frustrated.

When we look at ourselves, we have to learn how to love and admire what is good about us, and not go back to the negative feelings we had in our childhoods.

We can accept ourselves, even if others do not. We can be our own loving parents.

　　　　　FATIGUE FREE MADE CRYSTAL CLEAR!

Chapter 13

Energy Stabilizer Meditation

THERE ARE SOME things you can do on your own. I'll describe a morning meditation and an evening meditation to keep your energy stabilized, to get prepared for, and get over, toxic interactions.

Morning Grounding Meditation

The morning is good time to prepare, to ground yourself. Find a quiet place where you won't be interrupted for at least ten minutes. Sit on the floor or a favorite cushion. "Grounding" is on the ground.

Before starting, close your eyes for a few minutes and describe a positive intention for the day, what you would like to have happen, set Your Positive Daily Intention.

Take five deep breaths, breathing in through your nose, exhaling slowly through pursed lips, through your mouth.

If you wish, listen to some peaceful background music, music that helps you feel calm and relaxed.

Imagine, while you are sitting there, white light at the top of your head. Perhaps it is divine, let it be what it means for you. That energy trickles down from the crown of you head (the crown chakra), like raindrops though the head past your "third" eye, down through your neck, down through your chest, down in a trickle through your heart chakra, as you breathe, through your stomach area and your back evenly, while you continue breathing slowly in through your nose and exhaled through your mouth.

Meanwhile, the energy flow is helping any part of your body that needs soothing energy.

Continue the energy flow from stomach to thighs, soothing and releasing anything that is tense and not peaceful, down to your knees, trickling down to your calves, slowly, to your ankles and your feet, finally to the soles of your feet.

As you breathe, imagine this divine light releasing any tension, replacing it with love, pure love, as it flows from the tip of your head to your soles and then to Mother Earth.

You are releasing this way anything that is not serving your highest good, with the loving, divine light, flowing through your body, purifying you, filling your body from the inside out with pure, positive, divine loving energy.

Do this daily for 5 to 10 minutes, getting toxic elements released, transmitted out of your body and to the Earth.

This energy meditation will help you be more focused and centered throughout the day. You will notice that you will attract more positive, more loving people on a daily basis. Like attracts like. As you become more loving, you will attract more loving people.

You will see huge changes in your life soon after you begin this daily practice.

Evening Meditation

At the end of the day, you will want an Evening Meditation, to ground out and clear out everything you have taken on from the world around you, from the toxic energy from other people. Again, take only 5 to 10 minutes.

Find a quiet place, on the floor or ground, with a pillow or cushion if you wish. You may choose to listen to some peaceful music.

Concentrate on your feet, your foot chakra, and imagine energy coming up from your feet, from Mother Earth. Imagine a ball of light within you, starting at the feet. Take three deep breaths and imagine this ball of light exploding. It disrupts any toxic energies you have taken on during the day.

We are going to bring helpful light/energy from your feet all the way through your body and out the top of your head. From your feet, move the light through your legs, all the way to the chakra in the lower part of your stomach, dissolving energy throughout as it moves to your head.

The third chakra is near the navel, the belly button. Imagine the light to come here and the ball of light exploding, again, transmitting beneficial energy throughout your body and out of the top of your head.

The next chakra is in the middle of your chest. Continue to breathe, as you imagine a ball of light near your heart, exploding, fragmenting any toxic elements, and then picture this energy passing up through your body, out the top of your head.

Next chakra is in your neck area, and again have your ball of light go there, explode, pulverizing the problem elements, then moving them through and out the top of your head.

Your third eye is chakra six, your "third eye" in the middle of your forehead, and you'll do as before, having the ball of light explode and carry away the toxic elements, flowing out the top of your head.

Your crown chakra, at the top of your head, seems to experience an exploding ball of light, as you take two deep breaths, forcing out toxic energy trough the top of your head, picturing a white, divine fountain of light.

This meditation releases what you have picked up through the day that is not in your best interest.

Continue this meditation for 5-10 minutes a day, from the soles of your feet to the top of your head, and you will feel more peaceful at night, prepared for sleep and for the next day. You will be more centered, focused. The commitment to this will help you rid yourself of energy that is not yours, picked up from others during the day.

[This chapter appeared originally in my first book, *PAIN FREE,* also published by Outskirts Press and available from Outskirts, Amazon, and Barnes & Noble.]

                    FATIGUE FREE MADE CRYSTAL CLEAR!

Testimonials

[These include some testimonials also presented in *PAIN FREE and FEAR FREE and HAPPINESS, my* first three books. These are not limited to the increase of happiness, and they have had minor editing, primarily to preserve the privacy of their writers.]

WOW! I woke up this morning thinking about you and your incredible work that you do. I had a private session with you about a year ago. It was only 30 minutes but it was without a doubt very, very powerful. It made me a believer in what you do, I was a total skeptic before the session. Not now, I knew within 24 hours after our session that something was shifting, physically, in a good way. Unfortunately, I didn't keep up with listening to the MP3's that were included in the package that I purchased and now I'm back to where I started. The package was purchased from Eram Saeed's webcast called From Heartache to Joy. FHTJ.com. I truly wish that I had recorded our session so that I could replay it over and over. Dawn, you're a remarkable woman. Thank you for changing my life for the better! I pray that you are showered with Blessings everyday of your life. You certainly deserve it! P.S. I have no affiliation with Eram Saeed what so ever.

J

Last year I purchased Dawn Crystal's Anti-Aging set of mp3s from Your Wealth Revolution and a 30-minute phone session was also included. I was able to talk to Dawn in early September, and although I mainly wanted to ask about help for weight gain, I'm glad I mentioned to her that I experienced a kind of numbness and ache in my left arm when lying down. It was probably something impeding the circulation, but using her special sounds and breath work, Dawn worked on the problem, and later that night when I went to sleep, I noticed that there was a definite improvement. Subsequently the symptoms disappeared. I don't know how serious the issue was but I'm grateful for being able to receive my first live healing.

Thanks a lot. Wish you all the best!

V

Hi Dawn,

I have a question about purchasing your healing mp3s. I'm new to purchasing these and wanted to know what the process

Is once you buy online. Do you receive the link or files through email and are you able to download them onto an iPhone or iPad?

My mom and I have recently discovered you and have experienced so much healing already. My deep appreciation for the work you do.

Thank you in advance for your help,

H

Hi Dawn, This is me, dancing with Joy. I had deliberately waited to get my Pupp's bloodwork repeated to give his Healing time to process. I Knew we would get Good News and we Did! His white blood cell count & lymphocytes are Normal! His blood platelet count went from 75,000/80,000 (low) to 305,000, gloriously Normal! It feels to me that our bond together has deepened as well.

My hip and lower back pain are Gone! I have now found an affordable Handiman that I believe will do a great job, allowing me to (finally!) put my home on the market. The fatigue persists, which makes me wonder what Lesson I have yet to learn or remember, or, what past Life issue may be raising up for healing. I may be making another appointment with you.

Your humbleness, clear Intent and Focus on Only that which is to the Highest, Greatest Good, and determination that no ego only Source is what is are Inspiring and humbling. I So Appreciate and am Grateful to you and Source. I hope your Pupp's leg is All Better! Congratulations on & many Blessings in your new Home!

From Zorro & my Hearts to Yours,

Thank you! Thank you! Thank you!

Love, B

I have sought out and have paid so many sound healers and nothing shifted for me.

Until I heard a radio show Dawn Crystal was doing. Something shifted for me by just listening to the replay of this radio show. Dawn Crystal is the real deal and definitely sent to us by the Divine. I booked a session, I was somewhat skeptical but my intuition said do it, loud and clear.

It was amazing. Dawn shared that the process would be working for awhile after my session. It's been two weeks today and I have not felt this joyous and free in 20 years. Give yourself the best gift ever, work with Dawn Crystal, I will continue to work with her as long as she is doing this work.

Bless you Dawn. Your healing is a miracle.

M

Dear Dawn,

"Miraculous" is the word that keeps coming to mind as every day brings the Joy of discovering something else that has been Transformed. And each return to Balance feels as natural as Breathing!

I feel like I have come back to Life, Lighter & more Present with myself.

A back injury... Healed! No more pain! I had listened to the Joint segment of Total Body Rejuvenation ONCE and my hips are remarkably better. I discovered this as my Pupp & I were hiking in the park & I Felt So Much more Comfortable!

I was brushing my teeth when I realized that the tooth pain was Gone! We had worked on "fear" for literally a few minutes and, the next time something "scary" had happened - I Felt Calm, and the phrase that popped into my head was, "I Am Strong!", and, I Felt that!

And the Messages you gave me from my Beautiful Daughter who had passed a month before our Private Session have Transformed my Life! Yes, there are times I cry, times I would like to text or call her, of course! But now, the predominate feeling is one of Joy, of Relief - She Really IS OK! More than "ok", she Is Filled with Joy & Peace & Love, & is having a Grand Adventure in her New Life! I "knew" that before, now, I Really Know it!

There's more too, but I think the above conveys that Dawn Crystal IS the Real Deal! What it may not convey is your Authenticity, your genuine Compassion, and the Nonjudgmental, Caring ways you interact with those of us Blessed with meeting you and being Transformed through your Gifts. I am So Grateful for the Wonderful Changes you have, and still are, through your recordings, bringing about in my Life.

Thank You Dawn Crystal. Many Blessings to You!

Love,

B

Dear Dawn Crystal,

Your sessions are a great help for me, a very positive transformation is going on!

I always believed in the healing capacities of sound, and now you give me the opportunity to discover by your beautiful and powerful voice the incredible benefits of it.

I am very grateful for this magnificent present I received from you!

Thank you so much!

You changed my life!

love

A

Hello Dawn,

Yes, I would love to write you a testimonial!

I always feel at a loss for words just as the healing you do is beyond words. It is in the etheric and energetic realms that then transform into the physical. I feel more energy, liveliness, sparkle and joy in life.

K

Hi Dawn & or Dawn's team!

I'm a bit of an energetic being so I will do my best to put some of my experiences into words. You may need to pick out chunks for a testimonial. and I this is not at all coherent its ok to delete it!

I found Dawn through Learning Strategies. I was on the 1st series she did. I would have been on more, but somehow, I didn't know she did more than one. It was wonderful. I had hip pain when I slept, and the 1st time I listened while I was listening my hip pain went away. That blew me away! I listened to them intermittently, and enjoyed it. It made a huge shift in my relationship with my husband. I used it to clear issues with my dog. I do a lot of other energy clearing stuff so I got side track. I was always curious but never ambitions enough to look up Dawn on the internet until about February. I was out on a bike trail with the dogs & slipped on ice & broke my leg. I had a lot of down time so I looked her up. I was looking online for a private session. On like how did I create this how can I uncreate this what else is possible? And what can I clear so it doesn't happen in the future? That kind of looked like a dead-end street, but I signed up for her email.

So, with the Total Body Rejuvenation I kept listening to the Ankle one a lot. I do think it has helped the healing process. I have also listened

   FATIGUE FREE MADE CRYSTAL CLEAR!

to the teeth one & that has been great. I've unfortunately had a lot of dental work a & had to have 2 crowns this winter as well & it has been wonderful!

I got the new dental package as well & the coolest thing about that is that my teeth feel cleaner after I listen to it. I also had a tooth that had a fill that hurts & it hurts a lot less now. I still can't floss behind it but I have started chewing on that side of my mouth.

I have no desire to get sick but if I do, I know I can out one of your mp3's on & clear it which is phenomenal!

Do you of have you considered doing something on sleep? My husband has problems sleeping.

Thank you for being you & in the world & on the planet (yes possibly the same thing). Thank you for being as weird & wonderful as you are, and using your gifts & talents to contribute to the world.

And finally I just have to say this is really weird. This is probably the longest email I've written ever.

Thank you

M.

Dear Friends,

I participated on a free on line course with Siegfried. I'm sorry I can't recall all her name yet it was a gift indeed as she introduced Dawn amongst many guests.

Dawn was one of two who touched me very deeply in a short video where she used her ' sounding '.

This went so deep as if an invisible hand was reaching inside me and lifting out what was ripe to be released, in my case emotional pain.

Sound has always been a close friend of mine though strangely I can't listen to much music these days.

Dawn's sound expression though had a wholly new expression, very pure and liberating. I could feel her journey that she shared as this gift was given to her.

I would want everyone to be free from pain, and know that Dawn will be able to assist humanity to a new place of freedom.

Thank you.

J.

Dawn Crystal's Anti-Aging and Total Body Rejuvenation sound healing PDFs feel miraculous! A literal Godsend.

I only wish they could be used without headphones from a CD or cassette for less EMF radiation. (Cannot be used without WiFi/cellular connection.) Would use more often this way.

Thank you, Dawn Crystal, for sharing your spectacular gifts!

D.

HI Dawn,

Oh, My Goodness! Thanks to You and Creator, I FEEL SO Much Better about my Daughter's moving to Heaven! WHAT a Gift that is! Also, I feel like I've come back to Life. There are things that I'm interested in and will pursue. I'd thought of something that has been a challenge for me and both the phrase, "I am Strong!" with the feeling to match, just suddenly bloomed within. Every day I'm noticing something else that is Better. I am so Grateful to you for having offered a session with you as a part of your package with Greatest You Summit. That was an extremely Generous offer and I Do Appreciate it. From my Heart to Yours, thank you.

Love,

B.

Dear Dawn,

First of all, thank you for this beautiful gift you are sharing with the world. You are truly a gift!

I bought your anti-aging program from Soul Talk. What a gift, especially for women, to use sound instead of surgery. It's a groundbreaking work!

I come from a family of musicians so the work with sound, coming from Source directly, definitively felt it was my way.

I will try to explain briefly what happened so far (as my English is not so perfect).

I started with "Youth Elixir" for 21 days, as I have a very thin skin and lot of wrinkles (I am 67). My skin looks more firm. I feel that this it is the starting point to get rid of the wrinkles. Maybe the wrinkles are a little bit less.

One day I tried to listen also the one for hormones in the evening, but two on the same day was too much, as I do other energy works too.

I continued with "Thoughts and Feelings" starting on March 30th. It blowed me away. I felt the immediate shift and well being. Really, amazingly powerful.

I feel lighter and happier.

So, thank you, thank you, thank you

Much Aloha,

B.

Dear Dawn,

This morning I realized that the big two scars I have on my right food after Hallux Valgus surgery 5 years before were vanishing, after 5 years staying almost as they were at the beginning.

Also the overall skin of my body looks healthier and spots are diminished.

Thank you, thank you, thank you, again.

B.

You made my day! Dawn is BRILLIANT and POWERFUL! I am thrilled with Body Rejuvenation, Pkg B.

Much thanks,

M

     FATIGUE FREE MADE CRYSTAL CLEAR!

Hi Dawn,

Thank you so much for the work you are doing! I purchased your Total Body Rejuvenation Package on February 17, 2019. Since I have had vision issues since I was a young child, I listened to the Perfect Vision about eight times.

I had my yearly eye exam yesterday. The blepharitis I have been dealing with for years was mostly cleared. I have also had very dry eyes and now my tear ducts are working much better. With corrected vision the best my eye sight could be was 50/20 and yesterday it was 40/20. My Dr. stated that I was the only patient he remembers whose eye sight improved! I am sure it will continue!

Love this package!

Take/give care,

L

Dear Dawn,

Just love you and all your programs i have purchased 3 of your programs: Anti-ageing, GAOPF, Total Body Rejuvenation would love to have the one with the weight lost too.

I was very skeptical at the beginning but the more I listen to your interview I really resonated with your sounds healing.

All your programs helped me so much in my development and so happy to get them.

I have listened Item+1+Clearing+Emotional+Pain mp3 and all my unnecessary emotions and pain from my heart just gone.

I encourage everyone to have Dawn programs to help and see life more beautiful and with more confidence.

Love you Dawn thank you for your amazing work and for existing into my life.

Much much Love and Light from beautiful Dubai.

Best Regards,

A.

I have purchased Dawn's packages and had so many changes and tremendous growth. Her one on one sessions have been life changing. Literally. Thank you Dawn!

P.

Hi Dawn,

I sent one response already, but not sure if you received it, so here is another:

I stumbled upon Dawn Crystal when she was a guest speaker on one of the internet spiritual talk shows I subscribe to.

What a find! I began to listen to her anti-aging, hormone balance, clearing lower emotions, and healthy hair/skin and nails short sound healings. While visiting with friends in MA, one noticed how I looked

   FATIGUE FREE MADE CRYSTAL CLEAR!

younger and said 'You are turning back the clock.' I knew it was because of these healings!

Dawn is such a clear channel. I had the pleasure of having a short one-one-one phone healing that was right on target. She channels with great compassion and truth. I have recommended her to many of my energy healing friends, and consider her an active healing agent on this planet. I am very grateful for being one of the many recipients of her gifts.

I.

Hi, Dawn,

I can't thank you enough for the wonderful session I just experienced on Quantum Conversations. About 5 months ago I invited a friend to come live in my house until he managed to get back on his feet again. To make a long story very short, I think he and I are soul aspects of the same soul as I felt an instant connection when he moved in. The words home, safe, and MINE filled my head and heart. I am still determined to help him, but the situation has become so stressful because of his very expensive drug addiction that when I signed on to this webinar, I was wired tighter than a 24 hour clock on a 10 day spring. Needless to say the first caller represented me as well only with a partner, not parents. Tears flowed through out the webinar and now I am no longer cold and tense, but warm, full of love, and ready to tackle this mess I have gotten myself into once again.

Words cannot say how grateful I am for you and your abilities. I had a session with you last year and it has helped a lot. This one reminded me to get back to the affirmation I had been doing before everything went pretty much to hell in a hand basket as the expression goes.

Unfortunately, I am tapped out right now so it is not possible to purchase your package at this time. However, whenever this young man finally gets a job and starts contributing to the household, I do plan to purchase this one as I know I can use every one of your mp3's and another personal session as well.I send you much love and many blessings as well as my gratitude for pulling me back from the ugly place I've been in for a while now.

Again, many blessings and much love,

D.

Happy to provide a testimonial, Dawn :)

I discovered Dawn's work when she was the featured guest at an online telesummit, and after feeling drawn to her unique ability to heal with her voice. I purchased a package that included a personal phone session with Dawn and was immediately struck by her ability to quickly and accurately intuitively hone right in on challenges from my past without my having given her any details whatsoever. Included with the package were MP3 audio files that don't take up a lot of time to listen to—in fact, I listen to them during the night while sleeping. I've also purchased a couple of Dawn's books since our session. I'm glad to have learned about Dawn's fascinating healing abilities and highly recommend both her audio files as well as a session with her for anyone wishing to receive emotional, physical, and spiritual healing.

T.

    FATIGUE FREE MADE CRYSTAL CLEAR!

Hi Dawn: I bought Total Body Rejuvenation package. I was shocked by the immediate results I saw the very first time when I listened to Healthy Hair, skin & Nails. My skin was glowing and the nails looks like I had gotten it done professionally. My Knees are doing much better also.

Thank you very much for the personal session. You were so kind, and resolve lots of personal family issues coming from generation.

Love

C.

Hi Dawn, My testimonial in support of your Get Out Of Pain Forever Program. I listened to your Mp3 for Ankles, Feet & Knees for knee pain which just flared up, don't usually get that. I listened once a day for just over a week. By the 2nd day it eased somewhat and continued to ease. By day 6 it was hardly noticeable...it's almost 10 days now and the pain is gone. I didn't take any medication or use balms or anything else, just listened to your Mp3 once a day...I've moved on to the other Mp3s in this program and am also on the Anti-Aging..thanks for sharing your divine healing gift of sound. You are blessed.

W.

I have purchased 3 of Dawns programs and had a session with her. I cannot encourage anyone enough to participate in her wonderful healing love and beautiful vibrations. I felt so much energy and love from Source through her I was floating. Speaking with her I felt as I was talking to my long-lost sister. She is a beautiful wonderful, truly loving lady. I am grateful that she shares her beautiful gift with us. I am grateful she has helped me remove my blocks.

Many Blessings,

S.

Dawn Crystal is a pure channel, meaning she is egoless in her work. She fully allows Source to move through her to client unobstructed and unaltered by any human ego mind distortions. I found myself fully able to trust and therefore open fully to Source Energies. The next morning, I was able to walk down the stairs with absolutely no pain in hips or knees. Not only is my body healing, but the healing ripples from body up through my human mind, clearing out distorted thoughts, beliefs, mental constructs that caused the physical 'dis-ease' initially. I loved working with Dawn. She is so True and Pure in her work, her intentions and heart. I am so grateful for her assisting me in finding the 'light' I could not identify alone. Thank you so much, Dawn.

K.

I love you so much! You have given me my life back.

I'm one of your Tuesday night students with Pete B. Your work has had a profound effect on me. I can be reached at j******. ***.

Thank you and I hope to hear from you.

Dear Dawn,

Many thanks for the session. It was very helpful and powerfully healing. My back is a lot better as though I had a break in the middle of my
body (legs and trunk) and it has gone back as one piece and what you
told me about moving forward and my husband made a lot of sense.
And especially healing the lack of consciousness. I do feel more connected and centered and really trust that I can move forward.

M

~~~

Hi Dawn,

I am thrilled to have a private session with you again. My life completely changed as a result of our work together. With immense gratitude,

A

~~~

Thank You so much, I am so grateful for this mp3 of sound healing. It
soothed and relaxed me. I am truly grateful for the kindness and love
you share!

Namaste

G

~~~

Hi

I love your work & really feel & see the benefits of doing the liposuction
~~~

mp3 .... it's totally out there, weird & wacky, it's amazing! Far better than going for surgery, fillers etc.!

I live in the UK & we really don't get much sun. As part of your beauty & rejog packages, I wondered if you could do an mp3 for a sun tan without having to go to the tanning salon or holiday in the sun .... it sounds crazy but if anyone could do it you could. Hope you can help; this would be a huge success considering the size of the tanning/fake tan industry.

With Blessings,

M

Amazon 5-star review of FEAR FREE:

Dawn Crystal is an amazing Sound Healer! This is her second book and it is just as wonderful as the first! I have also had the good fortune to experience personal healings from Dawn through the Learning Strategies Corporation "Silent Clearings" program for 2 years in a row. Her next "Silent Clearings" program is expected to start around February 19 or so. In addition, she also has a wonderful website and I have purchased a number of her programs from there as well. I cannot wait for Dawn to come out with her "Complete Dental Health" energy healing program on her website.

Through Dawn, I have been healed of lifelong anxiety and panic-attacks (I am 50), as well as a painful back and right shoulder that have been bothering me for many years! She is truly amazing and a really wonderful person as well. I feel very lucky to have found her and I look forward to many years of Dawn's healing programs in my life. Thank you for everything, Dawn! You are a life-saver and you deserve every happiness! Much love to you always. You have a True Gift and I feel so lucky to have experienced your healing directly. Aloha! :-)

L

This work has been so potent that the quality of my voice has elevated and I am now a produced composer and singer.

My relationships are healed and I have overcome patterns that I thought would take years to work through.

The emotional releasing was intense, more so on the 2nd or 3rd day of clearing.

I did the whole upgrade and harmful environments, as well as liposuction.

My body is free from cellulite and varicose veins (which was absolutely not the case before this) and my skin looks and feels better than ever.

I am living a completely new life, feeling like a lighter magical being constantly surrounded by miracles.

D

Hi Dawn,

This is a testimonial for the 30-minute session we had. I was amazed at how quickly you honed into the core issues bothering me. Even though it wasn't easy to hear, I knew in my heart that you spoke the truth. Clearing the emotional issues you identified will no doubt heal my physical problems faster.

Thank you Dawn!

K

Hello, I have purchased Dawn's Weight Loss and Anti-Aging Programs, as well as have had a session with Dawn. In the session Dawn was able to locate the blocked energy in my body without me telling her where the pain was. I could feel the energy move out through my body, giving me more energy and feeling lighter. Through the years I have tried many healing modalities; none of them have worked as quickly as Dawn's has. Looking forward to another session with Dawn.

R

Dawn,

I purchased four of your products, but I got a session with only one of them (would have rocked to buy sessions with all of them). I had been using the products before my session, and they did help. However, the session with you, really blew me away. I have never felt light like that before in my whole life. Totally awesome. The information that you gave me during the session was also really beneficial and I can see immediate results with use. Everything you said was right from my higher self and I know it. That gave me a lot of direction and new-found sense of self. I feel more in tune with myself than I ever have and it's only going to get better. If this is what happens in one session, I cannot imagine what would happen in more.

B

Hi Dawn,

I would like to share with my experience in using your anti-aging program

                           FATIGUE FREE MADE CRYSTAL CLEAR!

the mp3s are amazingly powerful, I felt the change instantly after each time I listen to them and after a time of using them every few weeks I have a glowing skin and healthy hair, plus that I feel emotionally and physically stronger and have more energy through the day.

Thank you so much for your amazing healing.

Love you,

R

Hi Dawn: I bought Total Body Rejuvenation package. I was shocked by the immediate results I saw the very first time when I listened to Healthy Hair, Skin & Nails. My skin was glowing and the nails looks like I had gotten it done professionally. My knees are doing much better also.

Thank you very much for the personal session. You were so kind, and resolved lots of personal family issues coming from generation.

Love,

C

Hi Dawn,

I have not purchased any of your products yet. I do have some recordings from your old webinars. I especially love the energy clearing work that you do in the webinar and listen to it daily. I feel at a level of higher vibration after listening to it.

Thank you for sharing.

S

Dear Dawn,

I have bought some of your packages and I can say that your work is awesome! The recordings have helped me feel so much better. I have some serious issues with my back, but after hearing your recordings the pain has subsided, so I know it's working! You are a blessing and thank you for sharing your gift to help the world. I can't wait to experience my private session with you!

With much love,

P

Hi Dawn,

I just wanted to say that you are so insightful and gifted. You knew so much of my 'story' and quickly intuited who was draining my energy, where I was losing it, and how to stop it. You were able to see where I held stress in my body and released it for me. I say prayers of gratitude every morning, and I now include having known you along my journey as part of that. Thank you for your heart-felt intentions, and the clearings I received. I listen to your MP3's almost daily now, and can see how I am looking and feeling younger every day. I have truly been telling so many about you and your gift of sound healings. You are an inspiration. From one light worker to another.... thank you, dear Soul, for sharing your gift with us so beautifully.

I.

Hello,

I purchased Dawn's Anti-Aging program the end of the year; previously I purchased the Weight Loss program.

Have gone through all the package items for the Weight Loss and just a couple of the Anti-Aging. Wanted to say that I feel that I have more energy; old energy is clearing out which is awesome!!!

I had a session with Dawn in December from the purchase of Weight Loss. I need to schedule another one I purchased with the Anti-Aging program. After my December 3rd session, I had emailed asking about pets. Was told if ever book another session could share some of it with my animals....

Thank you for your time.

Blessings,

R

Hi dawn, my name is C*******, Thank you so so much for taking the time to do this awesome call, I am so happy and so grateful that you did record this because in the email I received it didn't have a time and didn't know when to tune in for it, I have listened to the replay and the energy was amazing!! Looking forward to the one-day retreat in February with Erma FHTJ, I will be there virtually, although live would be awesome I am sure it will be just as awesome to be able to listen in to you and all the others for a full day of clearings, activations and amazing knowledge and tools. Thanks again Big Hugs Love and Blessings

C

I worked with Dawn to help me increase my energy. I have always had an issue with an energy dip during the mid-afternoon. Dawn helped me clear what was holding my life force energy down. Since my session with Dawn, I am amazed! I have had a steady amount of energy every single day since the session. I don't need short afternoon naps anymore!!! For my work - this is awesome! I am much more productive during the day so I am able to end my workday earlier. Everyone in my family is so much happier because of this! Thank you Dawn!!!

Dear Dawn,

Happy New Year!

I have a big testimonial for you, after purchasing total body rejuvenation and anti-aging. I listen faithfully to them, and at night for your best sleep item! Now though, my computer has crashed and I cannot find them! Please help, only when they are not there do, I realize how reliant I have been, in their helping me keep in shape in body and mind. No one can guess my age and I feel great, but please advise if they can be resent as I do not want to be without them for long!

I purchased through Erma Saeed and Judy; I think!

Love and light,

S

Dear Dawn,

I am so happy to get your 2 packages: No more pain and Anti-aging. I was so hungry to listen and experience your all mp3.

I can say that all the pain of feeling and emotions and heart-broken pain just disappeared in a miraculous way. I feel so good now and I'm expecting more good things to happen… I'm able to wear a dress which I was unable to close the zip, my cravings almost gone… I look radiant and full of energy and I feel my face it is glowing and I'm happy to receive so many compliments in the office…or from people who know me.

I listen to the Clearing feeling and emotions mp3 for 5 days in row maybe 5 times a day and from the first day I felt improvement….it soothe my heart …. So happy for that…

I listen to your life story and your sincerity of your story and it has just amazed me the way you went through all your life… I am so inspired by you.

Thank you, Patty, Carry, and

Thank you, Dawn, for being part of my life.

Best Regards,

A

Sharjah, UAE

This is my 2nd session with you!! The session we had last night was incredible. I had to lay down for 2 hours. My head and body felt a buzzing sensation. It was also trance like. The work we did letting go of the abuse with my father was freeing in a way I never experienced before. I feel more love for him! I didn't realize how much I needed to hear that he was sorry for his part in our relationship. As for my husband, I'm seeing things differently!! I want to take back my power more than ever!! Dawn, thank you dearly for your love, support and healing!!! You told me a few times that I am an old soul with a beautiful spirit!! You said not to let it go to my ego, and it hasn't. My heart and spirit needed to know and hear that my light is bright!! It isn't something that I feel that I'm better than anyone!! I never felt better than anyone, in fact just the opposite!! I look forward to strengthening my boundaries in our next session! I need more confidence in myself in all areas. But especially "making it on my own". I still feel like a little weak girl in that area! I know that God has put you in my path; I am immensely grateful to him for that! Thank you again!! Can't wait for our next session!! I'm sending you a whole bunch of love to your beautiful spirt!! Big hugs too!!

J

Hi Dawn,

Here's my testimonial for wonderful experiences with your healing voice.

Please edit or re-write to suit your needs.

First, I purchased the Anti-aging Package. Then purchased Facial, followed by Pain Free.

I had chronic fatigue for many years. Have released, detoxed, healed with other healers and master's for many years but kept coming back. With one amazing healer, my fatigue was getting better but mild attacks came back. That's when I met your healing voice.

With the Anti-aging program my inflammation went away after listening for a few days and became more energetic to live with vitality every day.

For those that may have similar symptoms this really means a great deal.

My boyfriend had pain in his hand from joint pain/inflammation. He

                    FATIGUE FREE MADE CRYSTAL CLEAR!

purchased the Pain Free program and now no more pain and the inflammation are gone. Every time the weather pattern changed; he was suffering. This was a symptom which was hereditary (came from lineage). So, It's magic.

I also had a private session which I highly recommend for everybody as Dawn really sees the whole you, sees the deep core emotional issues and releases it heals immediately.

The Pain program, while it is specific to the pain of different parts of the body it is recommended for any symptom without physical pain. I feel the healing addresses whatever you may need both physically and emotionally at the time you listen.

I have been listening to these healings for a few months and my body tingles more profoundly today. I feel lighter.

An amazing healing method beyond Sound/voice, enabling you to reach the Source yourself.

.. .. ..

PS Pain Free - when you say pain free one usually thinks of physical pains. You should stress that your healing really focuses into emotional pains as well. I saw "scenes" leaving.

Another thing. Regarding your book, I have an account with Amazon Japan and without purchasing from them I cannot write a comment. So, I'm asking how this can be done.

I am soooooo grateful and thankful to have met you Dawn. Please create

MP3s for "eyes" and Immunity for all seasons and cold/flu in the winter season.

Mahalo with love,

H

The first time I experienced Dawn Crystal, I was sitting on a chair resting my chronically painful knees. I was tired and dosed off, but was suddenly awoken by one of her loud, high pitched vocalizations.

I began to laugh...NOT at Dawn (I did not question her sincerity), but because I was so startled! After listening to the rest of Dawn's interview and receiving her remote Energy Healing offerings, I got up from my chair, and noticed that my Knees did NOT hurt!

Did Dawn's Sound Healing help my knees, I wondered ?!? I ordered Dawn's "Total Body Rejuvenation" program to experiment and find out.

After listening to Dawn's Recordings, my Knees felt stronger, more stable, and Pain FREE! WOW!!

A couple of weeks later, I experienced another (not the first time) bout with Vertigo, Nausea and lack of Balance. I had a phone session with Dawn during this time, and she saw and cleared blockages in my upper Chakras, and Grounded me very deeply so I felt much more Balanced and stable when I walked.

Dawn also saw causes of some of my physical and emotional issues going back to my Family and lineage, and she helped clear them. I would wholeheartedly recommend Dawn Crystal for her miraculous Healing programs and personal sessions.

Besides Dawn's amazing Healing Gifts, she has great integrity and compassion, and humbly gives credit to GOD for any healing that others receive through her work.

MANY THANKS & MANY BLESSINGS to you, Dawn.

- N

                    FATIGUE FREE MADE CRYSTAL CLEAR!

The words seem empty to describe the profound impact of my session with Dawn. She has an amazing ability to listen to the soul speak and is guided by Pure Source. In my short 25 or 30 minutes with her I was able to heal 30 year old emotional wounds I didn't even realize were still there! The impact on my life has been a delightful effervescent emotional resilience that I was unaware I wasn't enjoying !!

Strongly recommend you enjoy any opportunity to do individual work with her, no matter what you may intend, she has a direct link to pure source that will allow you to have your intention attended to - yet not limited by your vision of what you need. An incredible experience to be able to have Source work directly with you, through her pervasive nurturing healing gift!!

- M

Weight loss program: Using the Mp3s brought much awareness to parts of my body and perceptions I had that were not what I wanted. These help to clear and reprogram old patterns. My 1 on 1 session was phenomenal. I felt much lighter as I let go of many attachments/chords!

MK

Aloha Dawn Crystal,

You are so amazing! I just happened to catch you on Quantum Conversations today and as I was listening you gave me a personal reading, like you and I separated from the show and had a cup of tea together, you are really to the point and down to business, made me cry, and I just look at you and see Hawaiian Royalty, an Ascended Master, and Lemurian Honcho! (and mermaid!) Plus, you are so beautiful and brilliant.

Wow, what a gift to get a glimpse of who you are, your photo is very powerful, and a healing tool! I wish I could remember everything you said to me, you gave me the gift of taking off a blindfold, you said I was wearing a blindfold and couldn't see who I really am.

I look forward to the unfolding. At the moment I am a poet, and here is a poem about you!

> Dawn Crystal
> ever insightful
> full of grace
> with a flower in her hair
> she rises above the ocean waves
> she resides in the mountain
> presides over the whales, dolphins
> mystic reveler
> bubbles at her feet
> she is alive
> freedom between her sounds
> the ocean vibrates with her
> momentum she is garnished
> by the leis threaded by all of her children
> she has healed
> for she is the great one
> that all man has known for many ages
> she smiles because she knows
> she knows.

Love you, F. D.

San Francisco CA. USA

Hello Dawn - I purchased your Weight Loss Package. I have been listening for several days (not yet a week) and I lost 5 pounds without trying. Also my right knee pain has decreased and I feel I have more energy. I also have realized a positive shift in my self-image.

Thanks,

- J

Hello Crystal,

i have very hard water at the place where i live not so nice to drink.

when i use you energizing water mp3 on it, it becomes much softer and more alive.

J., Austria

It has only been a few days and just hit and miss listening to the modules and I lost 4 pounds and 1" off my waist so I look forward to the results as I continue to listen to them more regularly. I am grateful to have Sound Therapy available to assist with weight loss!

=Thanks

S. E.

P.S. I look forward to more changes after I have my private session too!

I had heard Dawn several times on telesummits and, each time, I felt a strong resistance. Fortunately, I have figured out by now that resistance means there is something important for me there. Oh boy was I right!

My session with Dawn really blew me away. Everything she said was spot on and everything she did hit the mark; so much shifted in these 30 minutes! The positive impact of the shift was felt immediately on all levels – physical, emotional, spiritual, and it translated into a stream of "good news" coming through in the following days. In other words, there was a noticeable turnaround in my life as a whole after that session.

Although I bought the session as part of a weight loss package, its scope and impact were much broader. Dawn makes every minute of the 30-minute session count, without ever losing connection, warmth and compassion.

In terms of the weight loss package, I am still going through the MP3s, so it is early days. What I notice first and foremost at this time is a shift in approaching the issue and food choices specifically. I am quite confident that overall, the session and MP3s will translate into some positive results regarding weight.

I highly recommend Dawn Crystal. She is truly phenomenal.

V. M.

Hi Dawn,

I am in such deep gratitude to you and your amazing work.

I contacted you to work with my beloved dog and not only did he receive healing, I also got an amazing session with you! You are a truly divine being and for anyone that is looking for healing... Dawn is an incredible healer...

Lots of love and gratitude

N

Dear Dawn,

I purchased all your energy downloads and have been playing them regularly since summer and I must say, they make me feel at peace and full of optimism. We also had two one on one session which I enjoyed immensely. My life has become more of experiencing trust and lightness which I am so very grateful for. You certainly have helped lifting much burden from my shoulders. Thank you so very much for your immense support!

May the light guide you at all times, always, much love

C

Part of me felt kind of stupid and crazy for signing up for this even though I've been using your programs for decades. I mean, I can't exactly afford it, and it's just some lady making weird noises over the phone. But my intuition kept urging me, so I went for it.

I'm almost 50 but had such an excruciating childhood, I've still suffered the effects no matter how hard I've tried everything under the sun to heal. Some things have helped but not enough to quell the constant underlying desire to end it. I thought about killing myself all the time as a kid, and the desire always remained no matter how hard I tried to heal and think positive. I would never do it because I wouldn't leave my child alone in the world, and I knew it was just leftover darkness, but to varying degrees it was the backdrop to even the happiest of times for my entire life.

Well, yesterday was Suicide prevention day, and I realized that I had not thought about killing myself for several days. That weight is gone. There's light in that place. So, that's pretty cool for only one session. Thanks for that. I'm excited to see what happens next.

L

Dear Dawn,

Being an energy healer, medical intuitive, empath, animal communicator myself, I can truly say that you are very gifted and that your sound healing frequencies are very strong and effective.

I thoroughly enjoyed the private session you so generously included in the purchase of your total body Rejuvenation program. It made me feel so much better, more grounded and alive. But most important I could feel your passion for your work. You truly want to be of service and your heart connection with the client is very strong. It has been an honor connecting with you via Skype.

Thank you. You are an inspiration for me.

With Angel blessings,

A

   FATIGUE FREE MADE CRYSTAL CLEAR!

August was a particularly difficult month for me. Fortunately, I had my private session with Dawn on September 3rd. That session was phenomenal. I released much negative energy I didn't even know I had. That night, I had the first good night's sleep I have had in a long time. The dreams were positive, too, instead of ones about some tragedy or another that I had to overcome. I am currently working my way through the series of Abundance Blocks mp3's that were part of the package I bought and find them helpful as well. My energy is now more positive, and I wake up looking forward to how the day will unfold instead of thinking this is just another day I have to get through. Dawn is truly amazing. I connected with her energy during the webinar she was on and the connection became more evident when I spoke to her on the phone. You will not regret purchasing any of the packages she offers as she is sincere in wanting to help you and not just wanting to make a buck pushing a product you really don't need. She helps you find the true you that is part of the Whole/God. Once you find that part of you and learn how to allow what your desires to manifest instead of resisting those things you are attracting that you don't want, you will find your life has changed forever in a very, very positive way. I am truly grateful I found the one person who could get through my resistance and help me birth the part of me that is truly part of Source/God. Now I can continue exploring what is mine to do in this lifetime allowing only those energies that are in my highest good to manifest themselves in Divine timing. Dawn helped me, and she can help you, too, if you choose to allow that to happen.

D

I was in extreme pain back in the latter part of June/July. I do not know where it came from and why, and my appointment with Dawn was scheduled for July 21. I asked Dawn if she could move me up or squeeze me in because I was experiencing excruciating pain that I had never felt before. Since someone had rescheduled, she had an opening for the July 7, and I was able to take that spot. Dawn did what she does best with her sound healings and going to the core of the problem, I didn't even notice, but my pain went away and that next week, the pain was gone. It went as mysteriously as it came. It was miraculous. Thank you, Dawn, so much for your generosity and flexibility.

J

Dawn,

You're a magical gift to my life. Finding you randomly one evening after being guided in a dream by my grandfather who I channel with often, he gave me a perfect description of the person who I needed for my next healing. That very next day in my inbox I received an email that had a replay of one of your online talks, I knew immediately seeing your picture you where the exact person my grandfather had described the night before so I proceeded to listen to your free healing followed by purchasing the get out of pain package which included a private session with you. As I proceeded to schedule my first solo appointment with you, I was able to book my appointment the very next day which once again I knew this had to be more than divine intervention. My first solo appointment I noticed immediate shifts in my life so much I paid for a second solo session. I can't thank you enough for sharing your gifts with the world, your generosity at the end of my second session with a free bonus extra healing but more importantly releasing blocks that have hindered me for years.

You're a true blessing,

L

                                          FATIGUE FREE MADE CRYSTAL CLEAR!

Thank you so much for the information, Dawn. Today, I woke in a different world with a more positive attitude. You hit the nail on the head with the resisting. Unfortunately, allowing is easier said than done. I allow for infinite possibilities for infinite flow/abundance/happiness in my life every day when I do my chi machine exercise. I have been doing this for several months and I am still waiting. The resistance may be part of the shields I put up years ago when I felt I needed them to protect myself from verbal abuse, etc. Recently, I have been working on lowering those shields even though that leaves me vulnerable again. I am going to presume my subconscious does not want to let them go. I will work with more of the mp3's that you included in your offer. I know if I am persistent enough, eventually everything will work the way it is supposed to work.

Thank you again for the wonderful session yesterday.

Namaste' and aloha,

D.

Dawn, hi, it's Y****, the last caller from Monday's show. I wanted to write a testimonial and since I couldn't find where to submit it, I thought that I'd just send it to you here: Thank you, thank you, thank you! Those few minutes working with you changed my life completely! Especially in relationships. But most importantly, I finally feel the self-love that I couldn't before. I, for the first time in my life, feel deserving of love.

Thanks again, Much love and blessings to you,

- Y.

Hi Dawn, I was the one who was suicidal the other night when you were on Spaced Out Radio with Elizabeth Anglin. It took a little while, but as the night went on, I progressively felt better, and I wanted to thank you for that.

- L. M.

I am listening to the Live show right now....and I Feel Fabulous! Thank-You, Thank-You, Thank-You, Dawn Crystal....Many Blessings to you for the Awesome work you do!!!

- D. R.

Dawn, I am in rediscovery. The stranger that was my lost self returned to me by your powerful energy work. I feel clear-headed, balanced, grounded and in total amazement of the self I have to get acquainted with. I am ready for the new world that is coming at us with great speed--and your energy work makes me fearless of whatever the future may hold.

With heartfelt gratitude, and love,

- I.

Hi, Dawn, I had the honor to get selected tonight for you to work with me. I am S., living in ****, NC. I have to admit that when you started in with your sound healing, I said 'What!' I removed my judgment and just went with it. When you selected me for a brief session, I wasn't sure what to expect. While you were working on me, I felt light-headed. After a while, I started to feel lighter and more joyful.

Thank you!

- S.

Hi Darius,

I don't have an intention for this week. Instead, I just wanted to tell you that I bought a package that included a personal session with Dawn Crystal and it is the best thing I have ever done! To put it in a nutshell, I can't even remember why I wanted to work with her. (This is a good thing!). I found a list this morning of things I had wanted to address with her and was shocked that I had felt those things (fear, depression, etc.). They are just gone. Anyway, I hope you have her back. She is a true blessing.

By the way, if you use any part of this note for your show, please do not use the name on this email. You can call me Liz from ****** if you need to say anything. (No last name please)

Thanks, LP

Hi, Dawn, thanks so much for the session earlier I feel much lighter already and am looking to clear even more. I'm always so appreciated for your healing. It's really a blessing that you are providing this healing to the world. :)

- A.

I am so Grateful to have had my issues addressed...I slept so well...and

I have had a very rough 4 months... Thank You to Dawn Crystal for assisting me.... I felt so much calmer after the session...just knowing I was helped in some way

- K.

I appreciate hearing your story that you shared on Lauren's show. I just listened to the replay & the healing I felt was Amazing!!!Your courage to follow your inner guidance is deeply inspiring.

- C. A. H.

Dear Dawn, thank you so very much for the session yesterday. It was right on the money, and I really appreciate everything you did to clear me. I am feeling much lighter, and you really pinpointed some issues for me. I look forward to working with you again.

Take care.

- J.

Hello Dawn, this is J., the first caller on Monday's show. Wow, what an intense session that was!

My body was a rocking and rolling and releasing so much!

I feel like I'm still processing, and I haven't been feeling well (anxious, etc.).

Thank you so much!

- J.

     FATIGUE FREE MADE CRYSTAL CLEAR!

The winter depression has also lessened, and I was able to attend a family function that for years I had not gone to this time of year, and as well, my energy levels are up, which isn't usual for this time of year.

- A.

Hi Dawn, first of all, I have to tell you I absolutely love the work you do

and the results I get. I am part of the Learning Strategies Tues. eve. group.

You have been such a blessing in my life. In fact, I listened to last Tuesday's event again early this morning. I know I will sleep well afterward....

C.

Hi Dawn! I wanted to thank you for the healing tonight on Lauren's call! I feel so amazing! I did buy your Higher Self package and I have a session with you this Saturday. I did have a question in the interim; I know you mentioned healing abundance was part of one of the benefits of this package. I was also interested in your Wealth package too.

C.

Hi Dawn,

Wanted to let you know, following my session, this past Sunday, April 15th, I did keep focusing on letting stuff release and integrating higher frequencies. Feelings/emotions did come up and Tuesday evening I got shown and released at a deeper level than ever before an incident with my Dad when I was about 11 yrs that was still impacting me in a very limiting way. I immediately felt more energized, and more capable of 'doing life', creating what I love and desire; shifting from a "I can't" to a "I can" come from/attitude. YAY!!!

And as you said might happen, I did feel some aches/pains in my body following the session, however, that is subsiding. :-)

Thank you SOOO much!

And I look forward to our next session at the end of the month!

Love,

L

Hello Dawn,

Delighted to write a testimonial for you:

So many of us work between struggle and hope in our lives. I've been trying to manage anxiety, heal from physical ailments, while also wanting to grow into more abundance and higher energetic integrity. I have found Dawn's voice guidance and acoustic clearings to be enormously helpful and transformative. With dedication, I listen to her modules daily and also regularly journal. In only two weeks, I feel more attuned, expanded and wholly rooted in my own two feet.

Wishing you ever greater circles of influence, and much love,

A

Dawn,

'I've been meaning to send you this testimonial for a few days now but a funny thing has happened. I keep forgetting to write it because I keep forgetting I had any problems. (LOL) I only remembered now because I saw the list I had written before our session that said things like, "I am gripped by fear" or "I feel like my soul has been crushed". I looked at that list this morning and thought, "I was?"... "It did?" I can't even relate to that anymore.

It's taken a minute, but I finally understand why that is. Somehow in that session, it was as if I stepped through a thin veil into a slightly different version of me. It happened so easily and gently that I hardly noticed. The issues associated with the 'other me' have just fallen away and it feels like I have always been the way I am now. I know that sounds totally weird but who cares! I love the 'new' me!

I am so incredibly grateful for this transformation and the session. I don't think I have ever felt so 'seen'. To say you have changed my life for the better would be a meager understatement. Thank you, thank you, thank you!!

DP

PS - I also sent a note to ****** to let him know how great it was to work with you.

All the best,

D****

I have purchased three of Dawn's programs and had a session with her. I cannot encourage anyone enough to participate in her wonderful healing love and beautiful vibrations. I felt so much energy and love from Source through her, I was floating. Speaking with her, I felt as I was talking to my long-lost sister. She is a beautiful wonderful, truly loving lady. I am grateful that she shares her beautiful gift with us. I am grateful she has helped me remove my blocks.

Many Blessings,

S.

I have purchased 2 of your packages-Total Body Rejuvenation and Anti-Aging, both from the Erma show, and I think they are brilliant!

I think your work is outstanding and I have done much spiritual and energetic work. Thank you for your pure openness and generosity of spirit!

Much love and light,

M.

Dear Dawn,

Thank you so much for sharing your amazing gifts with me. I am so grateful for your time & effort during my 3 sessions (FATTY - Anti-Aging Package). You are truly one of a kind. Last night's final call session was amazing and releasing the soul (baby) back to Source was so right. He/she would have been attached to me for more than 26 yrs. Finally, now back with Source.

Much Love & with Gratitude,

W

Dawn,

I've tried quite a few different packages from different healers.

Your Anti-aging MP3s are amazing!

When I am listening to them, I can feel energy buzzing all around my body, especially at the top of my head.

After listening I feel out of space at the beginning, but later I feel more grounded. I sleep better, I feel better. I feel connected!

Your work is very important and much appreciated.

Much Aloha!

And Blessings!

T

Hello Dawn,

The Anti-aging program works wonders! Mostly all the wrinkles on my face have disappeared and I look ten years younger. I am still working on the perfect weight part, my cravings are less, and I'm eating more fruits and vegetables. My skin is now very soft, and I am glowing. I feel totally different. Thank you Dawn for being who you are today and for helping people, as we all deeply appreciate your work! Thank you so very much!!

C. M.

Dawn,

You have GREATLY helped relief the Pain in my knees and other parts of my Body, with your BODY REJUVENATION package that I purchased via Jazz Up with Judy.

I am SO THANKFUL TO YOU, AND TO SUPREME MOTHER FATHER GOD ALMIGHTY FOR THE WONDERFUL BLESSINGS :)

Looking forward to my 1:1 session with you on NOV 24th

MUCH LOVE & GRATITUDE

and MANY BLESSINGS TO YOU,

N.K.

P,

I have just listened to the audio of Money Issues with Dawn Crystal, and I found it very therapeuric and has given me a sense of relaxation. Please convey this message to Dawn for me and Mahalo for the much loved session.

Regards

J.

[Most entries edited for privacy, punctuation, and format.]

About the Author

Dawn Crystal, an internationally recognized Voice Sound Healer, Body-mind Intuitive, respected Intuitive Life Coach, Soul Reader, Medium, Pain Release Expert and Best-selling Author (*PAIN FREE Made Crystal Clear!, FEAR FREE Made Crystal Clear!, HAPPINESS Made Crystal Clear!*), is known as a **LEADING TRANSFORMATIONAL EXPERT** incorporating ancient wisdom for modern-day success.

Dawn is passionate about helping people clear emotional and physical blockages, so they can manifest from their higher selves, step into their full potential, and lead their lives and businesses in ways that align effectively with their souls' purpose.

Dawn helps her clients to release themselves quickly from pain, emotional and physical, and she is an active mentor for entrepreneurs, CEO's, and celebrities, helping everyone! Dawn is the "go-to" person to get out of pain fast, in minutes!

Dawn participates regularly on global teleseminars, radio shows and podcasts. Dawn was recently interviewed by the *Today Show, Dr. Oz, Rachel Ray, The View,* etc. Dawn hosts her own radio show, *Pain Free Fast & Easy!* on the News for the Soul Network. For the past two years she has done a live bi-weekly program at Learning Strategies Corporation of Minneapolis called, "Sound Healing / Silent Clearing."

Dawn's unique sound healing CD has been purchased by clients around the globe, and she is available on both phone and Skype, as well as for teleseminars.

Dawn lives a peaceful life on Maui, along with her adorable dog, Hoku.

Dawn recently published three books in this series, *PAIN FREE Made Crystal Clear!*, *FEAR FREE Made Crystal Clear!*, and *HAPPINESS Made Crystal Clear!*, all published by Outskirts Press, available in paperback and ebook formats from Outskirts and from Amazon (amazon.com) and Barnes & Noble (bn.com).

"I wouldn't change anything about my life; it's a gift," Dawn affirms, and she transmits this inner strength to those she works with, giving them a grounding, a stable psychological place abounding with safety and love.

"I wouldn't do it over again, but I am glad where I ended up."

Dawn Crystal Recordings

To see a ten-minute interview video with Dawn Crystal, go to
https://tinyurl.com/ybg3osgp .

To see almost 100 videos featuring Dawn Crystal, go to
https://www.youtube.com/channel/
UCTVOeWAA5eI0_5T4Eagcn7Q/videos

Review *Fatigue Free*?

Reviews on sites such as amazon.com help connect readers and authors. We would appreciate it if you would write a review, even a short one.